The Menopause Diet

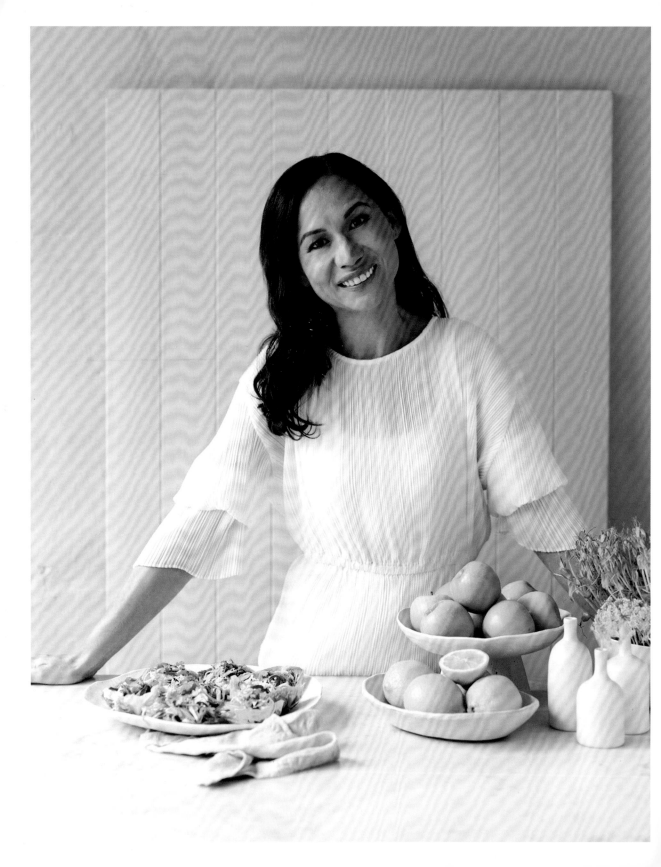

The Menopause Diet

75 recipes to reset the body and blast body fat

Nutrient-rich meals that support hormonal balance and aid in weight loss, plus tips and tricks for managing menopause symptoms and staying on track with your diet.

Faye James
A.N. C.N.

NEW HOLLAND

About the author

Meet Faye James, a powerhouse in the world of nutrition and wellness. With over two decades of experience and accolades including accreditation as a nutritionist and membership with Nutrition Council Australia and associate member of the Australian Menopause Society, she's a trusted voice in the field. As the author of the highly regarded anti-aging recipe book *The Long Life Plan* published in 2018 and weight-loss program and recipe eBook *The 10:10 Diet* published in 2019, Faye has helped countless individuals achieve their health and wellness goals.

Faye's expertise has made her a sought-after speaker and influencer, having collaborated with major brands such as Woolworths, Weight Watchers, Fitness First, and Goodlife. Her writing has been featured in top-tier publications like *ELLE, Body & Soul, Women's Health, Prevention, Glamour, Harper's Bazaar*, and many more.

Determined to make a real impact, Faye dedicated herself to solving a common problem faced by many women: weight gain during menopause. After extensive research and countless hours in the kitchen, Faye developed *The Menopause Diet* that helps women feel confident, energised, and in control of their weight. She speaks from personal experience, as she too manages her own perimenopausal symptoms with the diet she created. Faye was born in London, but now calls Sydney home with her husband, food photographer Darrin James, and their two children. With her passion for food and health, Faye shares her top expert tips in *The Menopause Diet* with the confidence that she can improve the frustrating symptoms women experience through this period.

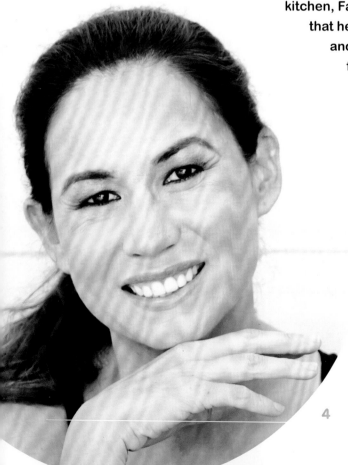

Contents

Introduction to the Menopause Diet

The menopause is a time of significant hormonal changes, characterised by a drop in levels of the hormone oestrogen. This drop can lead to a variety of overwhelming and frustrating symptoms including hot flushes, headaches, anxiety, sleep difficulties, irritability, and joint pain.

During the perimenopause and menopause, hormone levels fluctuate, triggering changes in the body that can have a negative impact on bone health, heart health, and brain health.

Additionally, menopausal changes are associated with weight gain, a decline in bone density and muscle mass, and an increased risk of heart disease.

But as annoying as the symptoms are, the good news is that simple dietary changes can help make this transition easier. What's more, there's no need for crazy fad diets or complex regimes.

A diet that is rich in anti-inflammatory foods such as fruit, vegetables, pulses, whole grains, olive oil, nuts, seeds, and fish can help counter stress in the body during the perimenopause and menopause.

Inflammation is widely accepted as the precursor to many chronic diseases and autoimmune conditions. Studies have

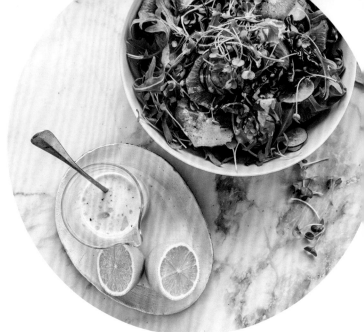

demonstrated that this kind of diet, akin to the Mediterranean diet, is effective in reducing the risk of heart disease and improving menopausal symptoms.[1] For example, a study published in the *American Journal of Clinical Nutrition* found that a Mediterranean-style diet was associated with a lower risk of heart disease, as well as improvement in symptoms such as hot flushes and sleep difficulties in menopausal women.

Another study found that a Mediterranean diet was effective in reducing weight gain, improving bone health, and reducing the risk of heart disease in menopausal women.[2]

These studies demonstrate the benefit of incorporating a Mediterranean-style diet into your lifestyle during the menopause. But science aside, let's not complicate matters. There are simple tweaks you can make which can not only futureproof your health, but also aid weight loss and increase energy and longevity.

In the next few chapters I'll explain how to make some simple tweaks to help combat weight gain, which foods to avoid, tips for keeping your gut happy, protecting your heart, maintaining bone health, managing stress levels, exercise and menopause, supplements and menopause, meal planning 101, plus my 75 delicious and fat-burning recipes for breakfast, lunch, dinner and snacks.

Combating weight gain

Menopause can bring about many unwanted changes, including weight gain. It's not uncommon to gain 2–2.5 kg over the course of three years during this time, and this weight gain can be attributed to a combination of hormonal changes, unhealthy eating habits and a decrease in physical activity.

As we age, our metabolism slows down and we tend to become less active, leading to muscle loss and a higher risk of heart disease and type 2 diabetes. That said, following these simple rules on a day-to-day basis can help combat weight gain during this period.

DO Eat enough protein

Recent research shows that eating enough protein is crucial for older women going through the menopause as it helps to combat muscle loss.[3] Aim for 1–1.2 g of protein per kilogram of body weight each day, which equates to 20–30 g of protein per meal. Good sources of protein include 200 g of Greek-style yogurt, one salmon fillet, or 200 g of beans (such as baked beans or four-bean mix) on two slices of wholegrain toast.

DO Watch your carb intake

Carb intake should also be monitored during menopause. A steady diet heavy in refined or processed carbs, such as white pasta and bread, can contribute to excess belly fat. Research published in the *British Journal of Nutrition* suggests that a reduced-carbohydrate diet may help decrease the likelihood of weight gain during menopause.[4]

DO Count calories

Calories should also be kept in check during this time. Your metabolism slows down during menopause and burns fewer calories each day, which makes it easy to consume more calories than needed. Eating out at restaurants and ordering takeaway should be limited to control portion sizes. Research has shown that eating three square meals a day, starting with a hearty breakfast containing lean protein and ending with a light dinner, can be beneficial for weight management.[5] However, restricting calorie intake to less than 500 calories a day is not advised and can lead to decreased muscle mass. Aim to eat somewhere between 1,000 and 1,800 calories a day depending on your height, weight and activity levels.

DO Try intermittent fasting

Intermittent fasting can also be a helpful weight-loss strategy during menopause.[6] This involves eating during a window of 8 to 12 hours and avoiding eating for the rest of the day. This approach is recommended for weight management at any age, but it's especially important during menopause. The easiest method is to eat your last meal of the day before 7 pm then have breakfast after 7 am the next day. However, it's important to check with a doctor before starting intermittent fasting to avoid any potential risks to your health.

Foods to avoid

Optimal nutrition plays a crucial role in mitigating menopausal symptoms such as mood swings, hot flashes, exhaustion, bloating, and potential weight gain. To maintain good health during menopause, incorporate my balanced Menopause Diet consisting of whole grains, fresh fruits and vegetables, and lean protein.

According to a study published in the journal *Menopause* in April 2019, a survey of 400 post-menopausal women revealed that those who had a diet rich in fruits and vegetables were less likely to experience menopausal symptoms compared to women who consumed more fatty foods and sweets.[7] Reducing the intake of these foods may alleviate the discomfort associated with the menopausal transition and contribute to overall health in the long term.

Here are my recommendations for the top foods to avoid.

DON'T Eat processed foods

Avoid potato chips, cookies and other processed snacks. They are loaded with sodium, added sugars and bad fats and can make you feel bloated and retain water. Instead, opt for healthier snacks like carrots with hummus, or seeded crackers with peanut butter.

DON'T Eat spicy foods

Spice up your life, but be careful with that hot sauce. Foods that are high on the heat scale can trigger hot flashes, sweating, and flushing. Stick to mild spices like basil, cumin, coriander, and turmeric, which will still add flavour without heat.

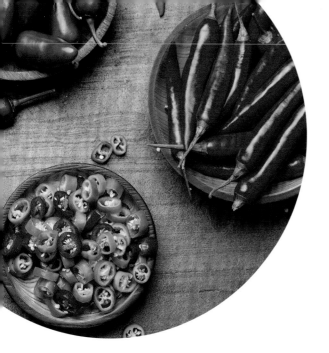

DON'T Drink too much caffeine

Love your morning coffee? It could be making your menopause symptoms worse. A study conducted by Mayo Clinic found that menopausal women who consumed caffeine were more likely to have hot flashes.[9] Try switching to caffeine-free drinks like hot ginger or peppermint tea, or if you need a pick-me-up, go for a quick walk.

DON'T Eat too much fatty meat

High in saturated fat, fatty meats like brisket and bacon can lower serotonin levels, leading to feelings of anger, grumpiness and irritability. Choose leaner cuts of meat like chicken, turkey or lean ground beef instead.

DON'T Eat fast food

Convenient, but not always the healthiest, fast food is often high in fat, which increases your risk for heart disease, a condition women are already more susceptible to after menopause. Choose healthier options, like a grilled chicken sandwich on a wholegrain bun, or have quick and healthy food on hand by packing lunch or freezing leftovers.

DON'T Overindulge in alcohol

While it's fine to have the odd drink, it's best to keep it moderate. It is recommended that women limit themselves to one alcoholic drink or less per day. Heavy drinking increases your risk for breast cancer and cardiovascular disease. Plus, research has shown that alcohol can trigger hot flashes in some women.[8]

Keeping the gut happy

During menopause, we can experience mood swings. One of the key factors in keeping our mood in check is to keep the gut happy.

Gut health is an essential component of overall health, and it is estimated that 90 per cent of the 'happy hormone' serotonin lives in the gut.

A healthy gut is home to a diverse community of beneficial microbes, also known as gut flora, which play a crucial role in regulating digestive function, immune response, and mental health.

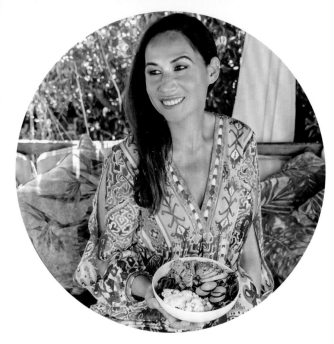

To support gut health during menopause, it is essential to eat a varied diet rich in fibre, prebiotic foods, probiotic foods, and foods containing polyphenols.

DO Eat a diet rich in fibre
Fibre is crucial for promoting regular bowel movements and supporting the growth of beneficial bacteria. High fibre foods include whole grains, fruit, vegetables and legumes.

DO Eat plenty of prebiotic foods
Prebiotic foods are non-digestible carbohydrates that feed the beneficial bacteria in your gut. Examples of prebiotic foods include onions, garlic, asparagus, and lentils.

DO Eat plenty of probiotic foods
Probiotic foods are foods that contain live micro-organisms that can improve the balance of gut flora. Examples of probiotic foods include yogurt, kefir, sauerkraut, kimchi, and kombucha.

DO Eat a diet rich in polyphenols.
Polyphenols are plant compounds that have been shown to support the growth of beneficial bacteria in the gut. Foods high in polyphenols include berries, nuts, and seeds. Incorporating these gut-friendly foods into your diet can help support the health of your gut during menopause, promoting good digestion, a healthy immune system, and positive mood and emotional wellbeing.

It is also essential to avoid foods that can negatively impact gut health, such as highly processed foods, sugar and excessive amounts of alcohol.

Protecting your heart
To protect your heart during and after menopause, it is important to focus on a healthy diet that can reduce the risks associated with the drop in oestrogen levels. Oestrogen has cardio-protective properties, so a decrease in its levels increases the risk of heart disease. A reduction in oestrogen also causes an increase in LDL cholesterol, which is considered the 'bad' type of cholesterol. However, by making certain dietary

changes, you can reduce these risks and protect your heart.

DO Replace foods high in saturated fat

Replace red and processed meat, butter, full-fat dairy products, cakes, and biscuits, with foods high in unsaturated fats, such as olive oil, avocados, nuts and seeds. Include at least one weekly serving of oily fish, such as salmon, sardines, and mackerel to provide essential omega-3 fatty acids that are beneficial for heart health.

DO Increase your fibre intake

Include a variety of fruits, vegetables, wholegrains, pulses, nuts, and seeds in your diet. Oats and barley are particularly beneficial as they contain beta-glucan, which has been shown to lower LDL chol-esterol levels.[10] Aim for at least 3 g of fibre per day, which can be achieved by having 30 g of oats or 250 ml of oat milk. Eating a small handful of nuts, such as almonds or walnuts, on a daily basis has also been shown to lower cholesterol levels.[11]

DO Consume at least five portions of fruit and vegetables per day

This will provide essential vitamins, minerals, fibre, and phytonutrients that help protect your heart. Choose wholegrain options such as wholegrain bread, oats, rice and pasta, as they have been shown to reduce the risk of heart disease.[12]

DO Incorporate soy-based foods

Soy foods such as tofu, tempeh, edamame beans and soy milk/yogurt can help reduce blood cholesterol levels.

DO Reduce your daily salt intake to less than 6 g.

This is important not only for heart health, but also for maintaining healthy kidneys. Research has shown that menopausal women can become more sensitive to salt.[13]

Maintaining bone health

To maintain bone health, it is important to consume a balanced diet that includes the right amount of nutrients.

According to research, up to 20 per cent of bone density can be lost in the five to seven years after menopause due to declining levels of oestrogen, which helps protect bone strength.[14] To slow this loss, it is recommended to engage in regular weight-bearing exercise and consume adequate amounts of calcium, vitamin D, protein, magnesium, phosphorus, and vitamin K.

DO Consume calcium-rich foods

Calcium is essential for maintaining strong bones and it is recommended to consume 700 mg of calcium per day. This can be achieved through consuming three servings of dairy or fortified plant milk (200 ml), hard cheese (30 g), dairy or fortified plant yogurt (150 g), calcium-set tofu (100 g), tinned sardines (60 g), ready-to-eat dried figs (four) or cooked kale (¼ cup). It is generally not necessary to take calcium supplements on top of a healthy balanced diet.

DO Consume vitamin D rich foods

Vitamin D is also important for bone health as it helps the body absorb calcium from food. It can be found in oily fish, eggs, and fortified plant milks.

DO Exercise regularly

Regular physical activity helps to maintain bone density and strength. Weight-bearing exercises such as walking, jogging and weightlifting are particularly beneficial.

DO Avoid smoking and excessive alcohol consumption

Smoking and excessive alcohol consumption can negatively impact bone health and lead to weaker bones. It's important to limit or avoid these habits during menopause.

DO Limit caffeine and soft drink intake

Caffeine and soft drinks can lead to calcium loss in the body. Limiting your intake of these drinks can help maintain good bone health.

DO Manage stress

Chronic stress can lead to a decrease in bone density, so it's important to manage stress levels through activities like yoga, meditation and exercise.

Managing stress levels

Stress and weight gain are two common challenges that women face during menopause. The connection between the two is more complex than many realise.

Studies have shown that stress can cause hormonal imbalances that can lead to weight gain, particularly in the abdominal region. To understand why this occurs and how to address it, it is important to first understand the role that cortisol, the stress hormone, plays in the body.

Cortisol is a hormone that is produced by the adrenal glands in response to stress. Cortisol helps the body respond to stress by increasing the production of glucose and converting fats, proteins and carbohydrates into usable energy. While cortisol is essential for survival, when cortisol levels remain elevated for long periods of time it can result in insulin resistance and type 2 diabetes.

Stress-related weight gain typically occurs in the abdominal region because cortisol stimulates the liver to increase the production and release of glucose, which raises insulin levels and leads to fat storage in the abdominal area. This is particularly true in women who are experiencing menopause because the body is already undergoing hormonal changes, which can exacerbate the effects of cortisol and lead to weight gain.

The good news is that there are many strategies that women can use to reduce stress and avoid stress-related weight gain during menopause.

DO Get enough sleep

Sleep is essential for the body to function properly and reduce stress. Aim for seven to nine hours of sleep each night to reduce cortisol levels and minimise stress-related weight gain.

DO Exercise regularly

Exercise is a great way to reduce stress and prevent weight gain. Aim for at least 30 minutes of moderate physical activity each day, such as brisk walking, cycling or swimming.

DO Follow my Menopause Diet

Eating a balanced diet that is rich in whole grains, fruit, vegetables, and lean proteins can help reduce stress and prevent weight gain.

Avoid sugary, fatty foods, which can increase cortisol levels and lead to weight gain.

DO Practise stress-reducing techniques

There are many stress-reducing techniques that can help lower cortisol levels, including meditation, yoga, deep breathing, and guided imagery. Find what works best for you and make it a regular part of your routine.

DO Spend time in nature

Studies have shown that spending time in nature can help reduce stress. Take a walk in a park, sit by a lake, or go for a hike. The sights, sounds, and smells of nature can help reduce cortisol levels.

DO Engage in a hobby

Hobbies such as knitting, crochet and reading can help reduce stress. Find a hobby that you enjoy and make time for it every day.

DO Seek help from a healthcare professional

If you are having trouble reducing your stress levels, consider seeking help from a counsellor, therapist or healthcare professional. They can help you address

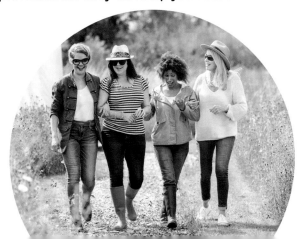

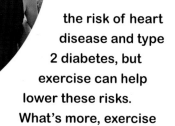

the underlying causes of your stress and help you develop a plan to prevent stress-related weight gain.

Exercise and menopause

Menopause marks a significant change in a woman's life but it doesn't have to mean sacrificing your health and wellness. In fact, using menopause as a reason to prioritise your fitness can have numerous benefits, from reducing the risk of certain diseases to boosting your mood. So why not embrace this time and make a commitment to take care of yourself?

During and after menopause, the body experiences various changes, such as muscle loss, abdominal fat gain and bone loss. However, regular exercise can counteract these effects and offer additional benefits.

Regular physical activity can help maintain a healthy weight, especially as muscle loss increases during menopause. It has also been linked to reducing the risk of various types of cancer, such as breast, colon, and endometrial cancer. In addition, exercise can slow bone loss, reducing the risk of osteoporosis and fractures.

Menopause weight gain can increase the risk of heart disease and type 2 diabetes, but exercise can help lower these risks. What's more, exercise helps boost your mood. Studies have shown that regular exercise is linked to a lower risk of depression and cognitive decline.[15]

While exercise hasn't been proven to directly reduce menopause symptoms like hot flashes and sleep disturbances, maintaining a healthy weight through physical activity seems to help alleviate these symptoms and improves your overall quality of life.

It recommended that you do at least 150 minutes of moderate aerobic activity or 75 minutes of vigorous aerobic activity per week, along with strength training twice a week. There are several options to choose from, each with its own benefits.

Aerobic activity: Brisk walking, jogging, biking, swimming, and water aerobics can help you shed excess kilos and maintain a healthy weight.

Strength training: Using weight machines, hand-held weights or resistance tubing can help reduce body fat, strengthen muscles, and increase calorie burn.

Stretching: Improving flexibility through stretching can be done after each workout or through yoga, Pilates or dance.

Stability and balance exercises: Improving stability through activities like tai chi or yoga or simple exercises like standing on one leg can help prevent falls.

Staying Motivated

Setting achievable goals, working out with a partner or friend, and regularly updating your goals as you reach new levels of fitness can help you stay motivated. Remember, you don't need a gym to get moving. Activities like dancing and gardening can also provide health benefits.

Make sure to warm up and cool down safely before and after each workout.

Supplements and menopause

Should you take supplements during menopause or perimenopause? I generally advise my clients that as long as their diet is rich in the right nutrients, there's no need for supplements. My recommendation is that if you stick to the Menopause Diet you shouldn't need to take extra supplements.

That said, there are some key supplements that you can take if you are struggling to meet your daily requirements through diet alone. If you are finding it challenging to follow the Menopause Diet because of travel or work commitments, then you might want to consider supplementing with the following.

Calcium

During menopause women are at increased risk of osteoporosis, a condition that causes bones to become fragile and more likely to break. Calcium is an essential nutrient for maintaining strong bones, and a daily intake of 1,200 mg per day is recommended for women over the age of 50. If you are struggling to get enough calcium you should consult your doctor but a supplement may be helpful.[16]

Vitamin D

Vitamin D helps the body absorb calcium and is essential for bone health. It can also help in blood sugar regulation and immunity. The recommended daily dose for women over the age of 50 is 600 to 800 IU per day.[17]

Magnesium

Magnesium is involved in many bodily processes, including bone health, regulation of mood and aiding restful sleep. It may also help with anxiety, joint pain and hot and cold flashes. The recommended daily dose for women over the age of 50 is 320 mg per day.[18]

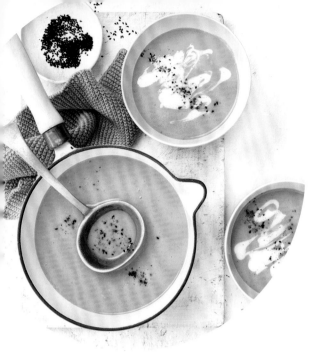

complex varies based on a number of factors but aim for 1.5 to 2 mg of B1, 1.2 mg of B2, 50 mg of B3, 2.4 mcg of B12, and 5 mg of B6 per day.

Collagen

Collagen is a protein that is important for skin health, joint mobility, and overall body maintenance and comes in either marine or bovine supplementation. During menopause, skin can become thinner and less elastic and joints can become stiffer. Collagen supplementation has been shown to improve skin hydration and reduce joint pain in some studies.[21] The recommended daily dose is 1–2 g.

Meal planning 101

I cannot stress enough the value of meal planning to aid you in your weight-loss journey during menopause. Meal planning can help regulate weight by allowing you to control portions and choose healthy, low-calorie options.

As outlined in the previous chapters, it's crucial you get the right vitamins and minerals to support your overall health. Meal planning can help ensure you get the nutrients you need by including a variety of fruits, vegetables, whole grains, and lean proteins in your diet.

The process of meal planning can also help reduce the daily stress of figuring

Omega-3 fatty acids

Omega-3 fatty acids have been shown to improve heart health and may help reduce symptoms of depression and anxiety when menopausal.[19] The recommended daily dose is 1000 mg of EPA and DHA combined.

Vitamin B complex

Vitamin B helps support the nervous system and can alleviate symptoms of anxiety and depression, which are common during menopause. It also plays a role in energy production, aiding in the reduction of fatigue. Vitamin B has been shown to improve memory and cognitive function and may also regulate hormones, helping to relieve hot flashes and other menopausal symptoms.[20] The recommended daily dose for vitamin B

out what to eat. You can plan your meals in advance and have a clear idea of what you will be eating, making it easier to stick to your plan.

Meal planning can also save you time and money by allowing you to plan ahead, shop in bulk and reduce food waste. With a meal plan, you can also avoid the impulse purchases that can lead to unhealthy snacking or ordering last-minute takeaways because you're too tired to cook.

Start with a list of favourite healthy foods

Make a list of foods that you enjoy eating, such as fruits, vegetables, whole grains, and lean proteins.

Plan for variety

Include a variety of foods in your meal plan to ensure that you get all the nutrients you need. Choose different types of fruits and vegetables each week, and try my Menopause Diet recipes that incorporate these healthy ingredients.

Consider portion control

Portion control is important during menopause, as it can help regulate weight. Use a food scale or measuring cups to ensure that you are eating the right amount of food.

Make a grocery list

Plan your meals and snacks in advance, and make a grocery list of the ingredients you will need. This will help you avoid impulse purchases and save money by reducing food waste.

Plan for leftovers

Batch cook some of the recipes on a quiet day (Sundays often work well) such as baked oats or spinach fritters so you can have meals over the following week ready to go.

Be flexible

Meal planning does not have to be rigid. Be flexible and allow yourself the occasional treat, such as a dessert or a glass of wine. The key is to balance indulgences with healthy choices.

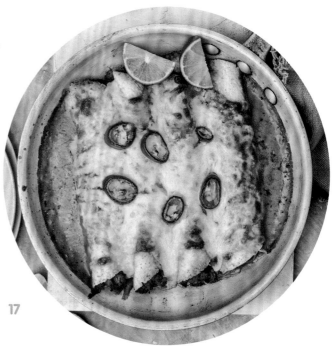

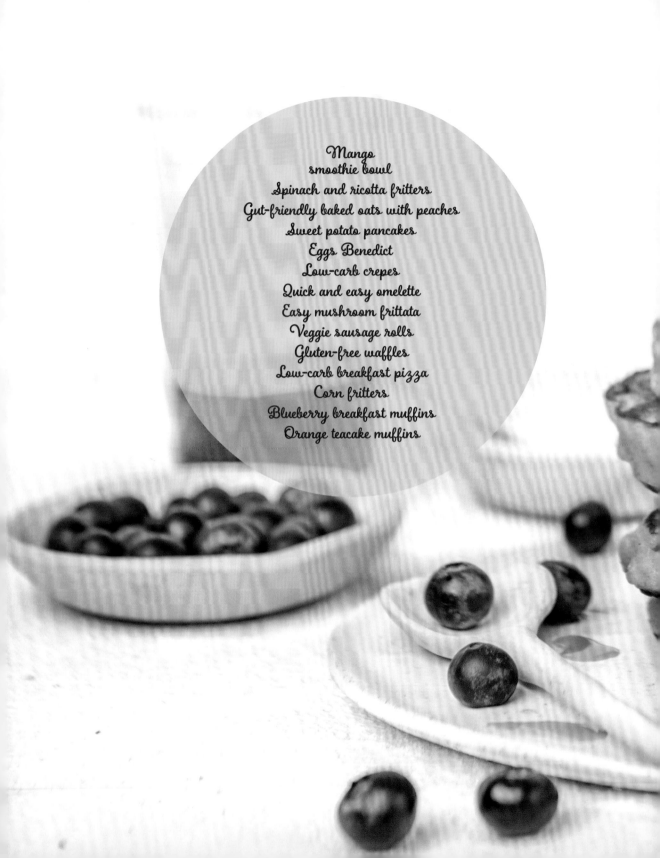

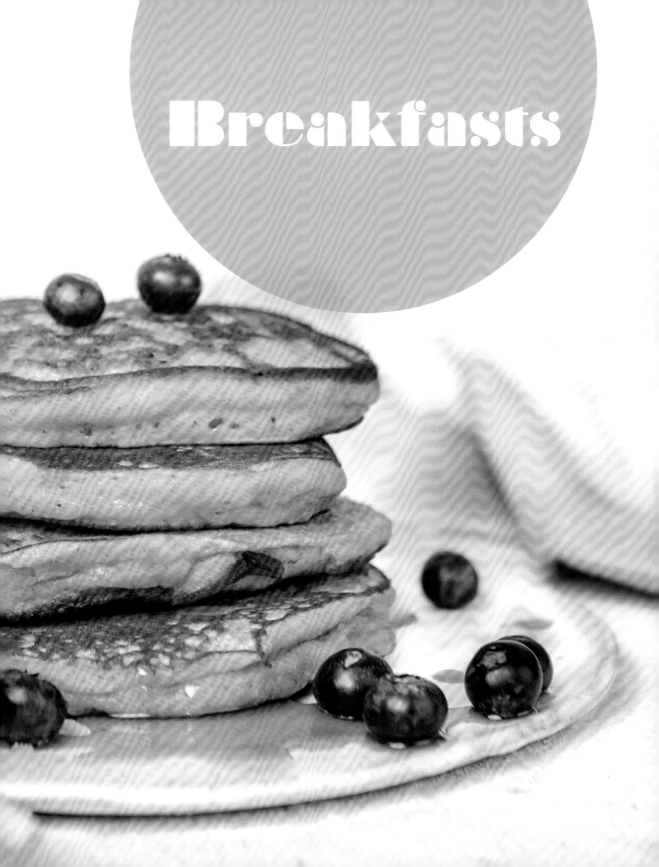

Breakfasts

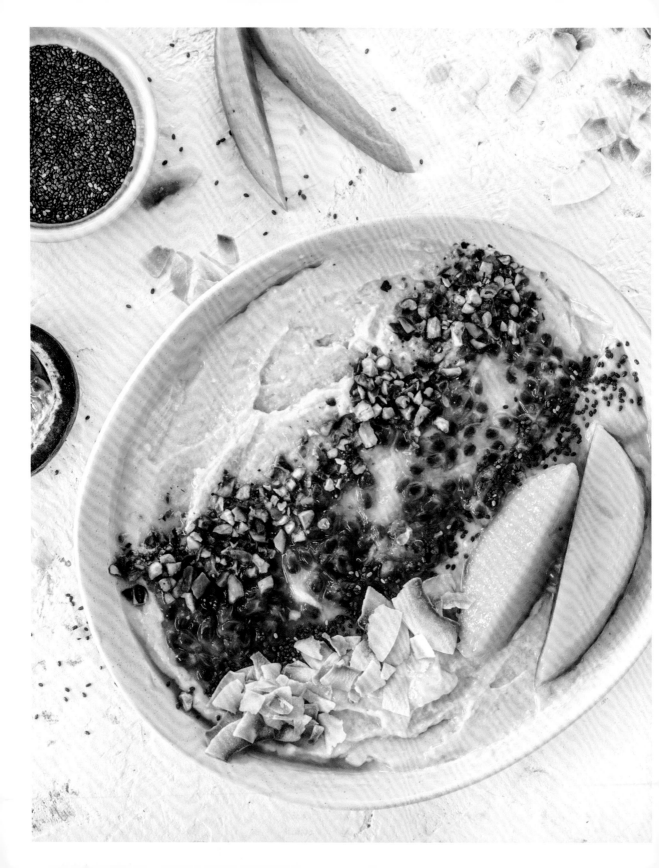

Mango smoothie bowl

Gluten free • dairy free • vegan • high protein • high in fibre

Ingredients

2 cups frozen mango

1 cup frozen banana

1 cup frozen pineapple

2 scoops vegan protein powder

½ cup coconut yoghurt

½ cup chia seeds

½ cup ice

½ a fresh mango, sliced

passionfruit pulp, toasted coconut and sliced pistachio nuts to serve

Method

Place the mango, banana, pineapple, protein powder, yoghurt, chia seeds and ice in a blender and blend until smooth.

Serve in a bowl and top with fresh mango, passionfruit pulp, toasted coconut and pistachio nuts.

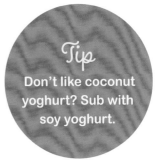

Tip
Don't like coconut yoghurt? Sub with soy yoghurt.

Spinach and ricotta fritters

Gluten free • vegetarian • low carb • high protein • keto-friendly

SERVES: 4–6
PREP: 15 minutes
COOK: 15 minutes

Ingredients

500 g ricotta

⅓ cup goat's feta

100 g spinach

2 garlic cloves, crushed

2 eggs, beaten

⅓ cup almond meal

salt and pepper to taste

olive oil for frying

rocket, cherry tomatoes and avocado, to serve

Method

Place ricotta, feta, spinach, garlic, eggs and almond meal in a bowl. Season with salt and pepper, and stir to combine.

Preheat the oven to 160°C. Line a baking tray with baking paper.

Heat a couple of tablespoons of oil in a frying pan over medium heat. Fry the fritters in batches. Spoon batter into the pan, around two tablespoons for each fritter. Flatten slightly and cook for around 2–3 minutes each side until crisp and golden.

Once cooked, transfer the fritters to the baking tray and place in the oven to keep warm.

Serve with rocket, cherry tomatoes, avocado and a drizzle of olive oil.

Tip

Want a vegan option? Sub the goat's feta and ricotta for vegan ricotta and feta and the egg for a flax meal egg.

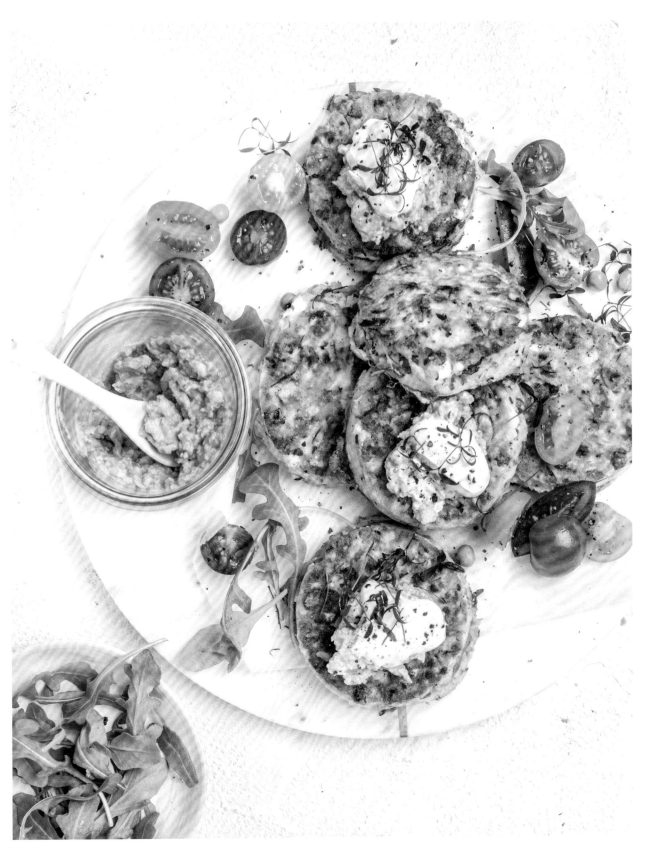

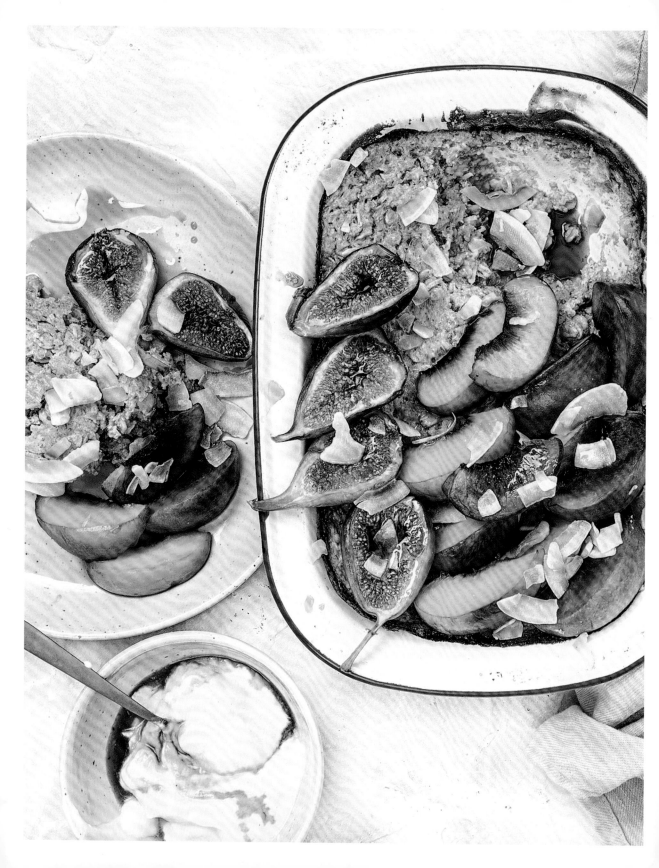

Gut-friendly baked oats with peaches

Vegetarian • gut-friendly • refined sugar free • high in fibre

Ingredients

135 g rolled oats

40 g desiccated coconut

½ tsp ground cinnamon

½ tsp ground ginger

pinch of sea salt

90 ml monkfruit maple syrup

1 tsp vanilla extract

730 g kefir

2 medium peaches
  or nectarines, cut into
  thick wedges

2 tbsp coconut sugar

coconut yoghurt to serve

Method

Preheat oven to 180°C. Grease an ovenproof dish.

Combine oats, coconut, cinnamon, ginger, salt, maple syrup and vanilla in a bowl then stir in the kefir. Transfer the porridge to the greased dish and bake for 40 minutes.

Meanwhile, place the peaches in a small baking dish. Sprinkle with coconut sugar, then pour over a third of a cup of water. Bake on a separate oven shelf for the last 20 minutes of the porridge cooking time.

Serve porridge topped with baked peaches (it's also delicious with figs) and a dollop of coconut yogurt.

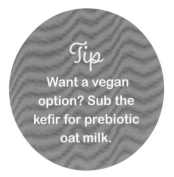

Tip
Want a vegan option? Sub the kefir for prebiotic oat milk.

BREAKFASTS

Sweet potato pancakes

Gluten free • vegan • refined sugar free • high protein

Ingredients

¼ cup almond meal

1 scoop vegan protein powder

1 tsp cinnamon

pinch of nutmeg

½ teaspoon salt

¼ teaspoon bicarb (baking) soda

¼ cup cooked and puréed sweet potato

3 tbsp oat milk

1 tbsp monkfruit maple syrup, plus extra to serve

3 eggs

1 tbsp vanilla extract

coconut yoghurt and blueberries, to serve

Method

Combine all the dry ingredients then add the wet ingredients and whisk until smooth.

Heat a little olive oil in a frying pan and place a blob of pancake mixture in the middle. Cook until the pancake starts to bubble and rise before turning over.

Serve with coconut yoghurt and fresh blueberries. Drizzle with extra maple syrup.

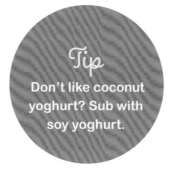

Tip
Don't like coconut yoghurt? Sub with soy yoghurt.

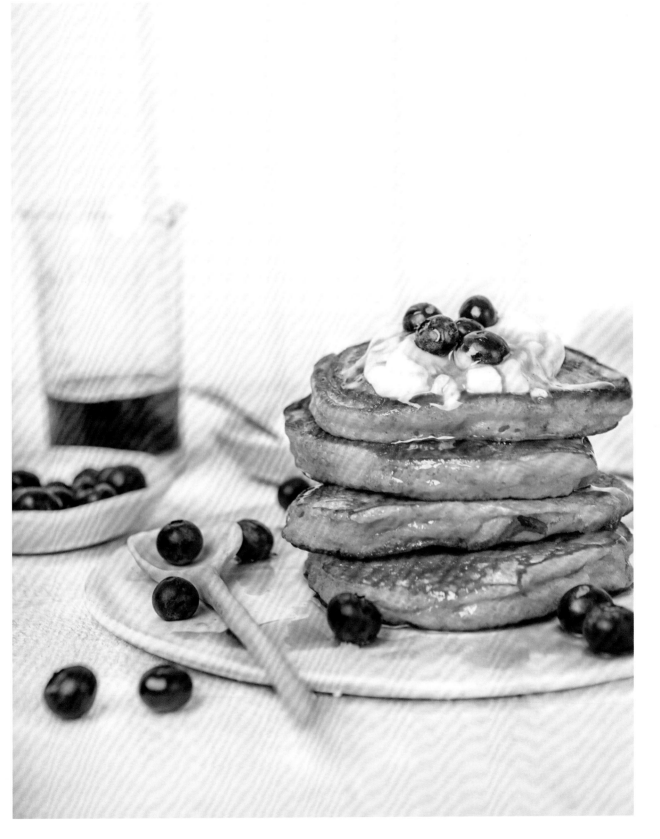

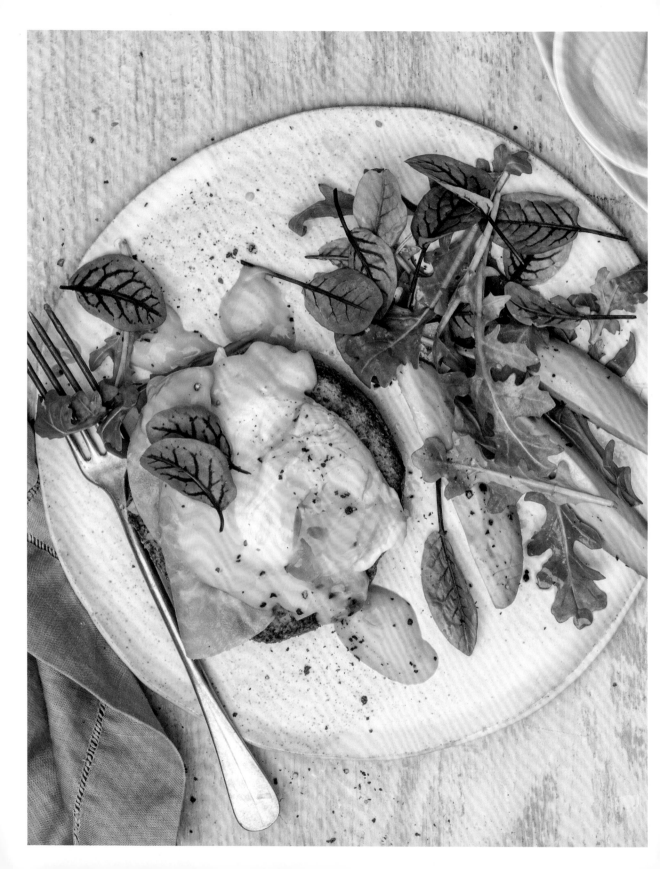

Eggs Benedict

Gluten free • low carb • high protein • high in fibre • keto-friendly

SERVES: 2
PREP: 10 minutes
COOK: 5 minutes

Ingredients

Hollandaise sauce

1 tbsp butter

2 egg yolks

1 tbsp water

1 tbsp lemon juice

salt and pepper, to taste

Eggs Benedict

2 eggs

1 tbsp white wine vinegar

1 tsp butter

2 slices smoked salmon
   or ham

Method

Make the hollandaise sauce by melting the butter in a medium-sized frying pan over a medium heat. Let cool and set aside.

Mix the egg yolks and water in a bowl. Create a water bath by placing the bowl over a pot of simmering water. Whisk constantly until the sauce thickens.

Remove from the heat and drizzle in the cooled butter. Add the lemon juice, salt and pepper to taste and whisk to combine.

Next bring a pot of water to the boil with the vinegar and let simmer before adding the eggs one at a time. Simmer for around 3 minutes before removing with a slotted spoon.

Place a slice of smoked salmon or ham on a toasted fluffy bun (page 141), top with an egg and drizzle with Hollandaise sauce.

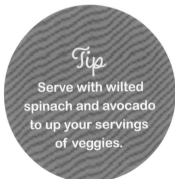

Tip
Serve with wilted spinach and avocado to up your servings of veggies.

BREAKFASTS

Low-carb crepes

Gluten free • vegetarian • low carb • high protein • keto-friendly

Ingredients

4 eggs, whisked

¼ cup almond milk

⅓ cup almond meal

pinch of salt

1 tbsp butter

coconut yoghurt, blueberries and monkfruit maple syrup, to serve

Method

Whisk the eggs and milk well in a bowl until light and fluffy. Fold in the almond meal and salt and set aside.

Melt the butter in a frying pan over medium heat. Ladle a spoonful of the batter into the pan and swirl it around to create an even circle shape. Cook for 1–2 minutes until golden brown.

Gently flip over using a spatula and cook for another 1–2 minutes until golden brown.

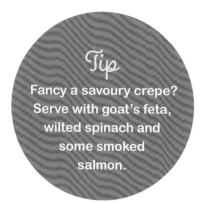

Tip

Fancy a savoury crepe? Serve with goat's feta, wilted spinach and some smoked salmon.

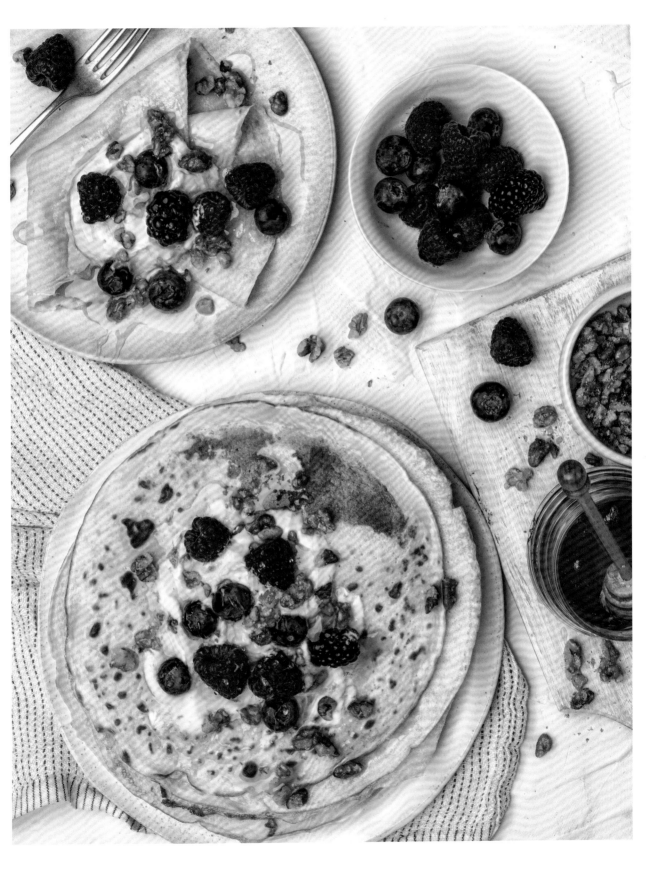

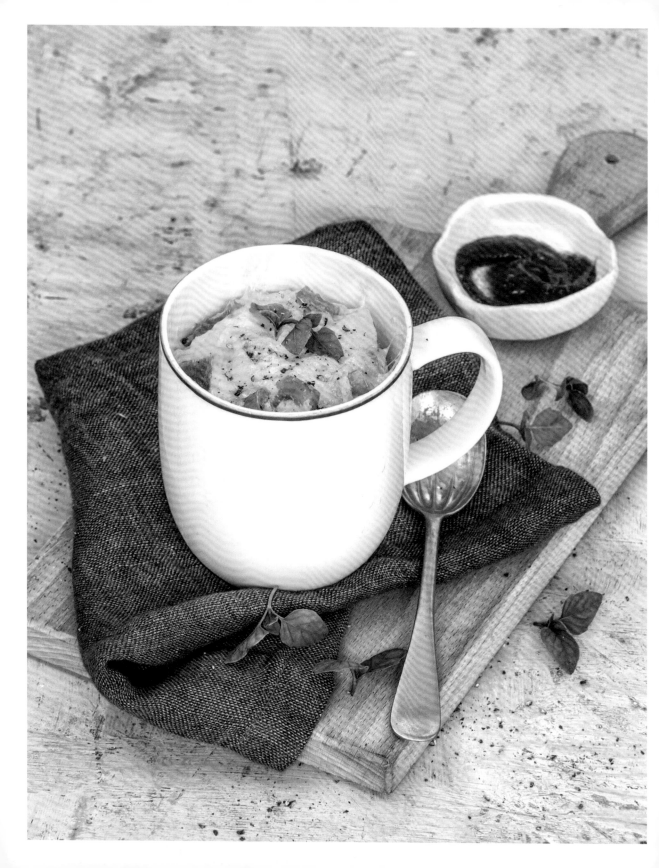

Quick and easy omelette

Gluten free • vegetarian • low carb • high protein

SERVES: 2
PREP: 5 minutes
COOK: 2–3 minutes

Ingredients

6 eggs, whisked

2 tsp soy milk

salt and pepper, to taste

2 tbsp diced asparagus

4 tbsp diced red capsicum

4 tbsp diced mushrooms

6 tbsp goat's cheese

Method

Spray two mugs with olive oil cooking spray.

Mix the eggs, milk, salt and pepper in a bowl and divide between the two mugs. Top with the asparagus, capsicum, mushrooms and then cheese.

Microwave on high for 2–3 minutes until puffed and golden. Serve immediately.

Tip

To up your intake of omega-3s, serve with smoked salmon, sardines or mackerel, plus a healthy serving of kale.

Easy mushroom frittata

Gluten free • low carb • high protein • keto-friendly

SERVES: 2
PREP: 5 minutes
COOK: 10 minutes

Ingredients

¼ cup sliced mushrooms

¼ cup almond meal

½ tsp bicarb (baking) soda

1 large egg, whisked

2 tbsp sour cream

2 tbsp water

½ cup grated parmesan
   cheese

a little fresh parsley,
   to garnish (optional)

Method

Heat a little oil or butter in a pan over medium heat, add the mushrooms and sauté for 3–5 minutes until soft.

Place the almond meal and bicarb soda in a bowl and whisk to combine. Add the whisked egg, sour cream and water and combine. Add the mushrooms and mix well to combine.

Divide the mixture between two small mugs.
Top with cheese.

Pop in the microwave on high for 90 seconds.
Remove and let sit for 5 minutes. Garnish with fresh parsley before serving.

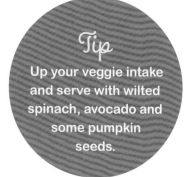

Tip
Up your veggie intake and serve with wilted spinach, avocado and some pumpkin seeds.

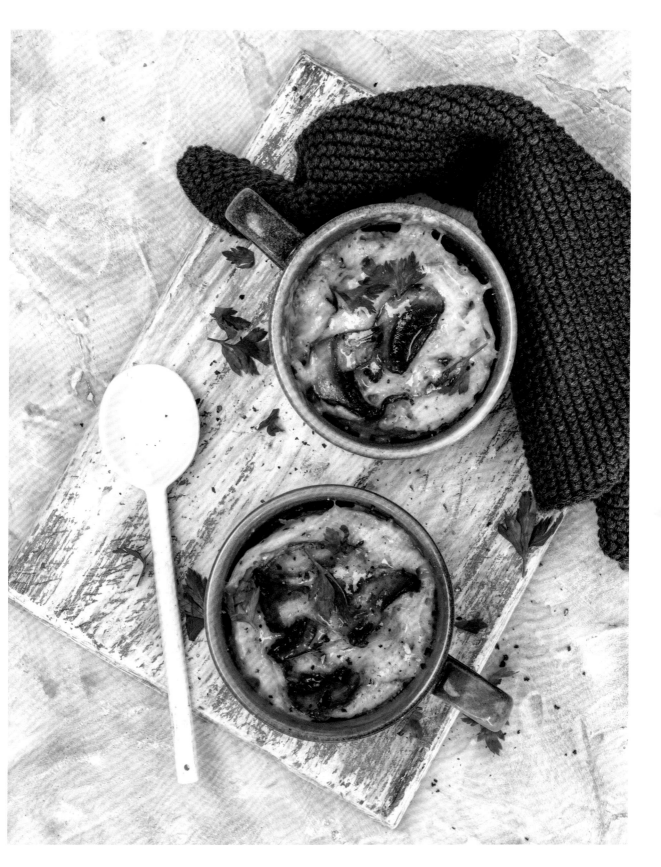

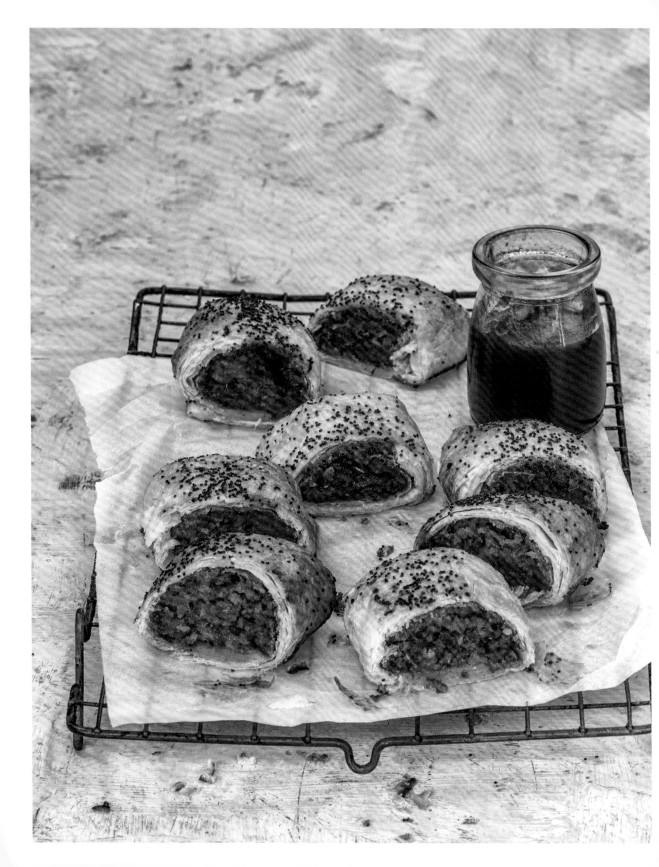

Veggie sausage rolls

Vegetarian • high protein • high in fibre

MAKES: 16 rolls
PREP: 10 minutes
COOK: 25 minutes

Ingredients

300 g sweet potato, roasted

400 g tin red kidney beans

1 zucchini, grated

1 red onion, diced

2 garlic cloves, minced

1 tbsp tomato puree

salt and pepper, to taste

2 tsp smoked paprika

1 tsp ground cumin

1 tsp ground coriander

375 g ready-made puff pastry

1 egg, whisked

sesame seeds, for sprinkling

Method

Preheat the oven to 220°C and line a baking tray with baking paper.

Scoop out the flesh from the roasted sweet potato and place in a food processor along with the kidney beans, zucchini, onion, garlic, tomato puree, spices and seasoning. Blitz until smooth to create your 'sausage' filling.

Unroll the puff pastry and cut in half lengthwise. Place sausage filling into the two pastry strips. Roll up then divide into sausage rolls. Brush with egg and top with sesame seeds.

Bake for around 25 minutes until the pastry is golden brown.

Tip

Don't like kidney beans? Firm tofu also works well in this recipe.

BREAKFASTS

Gluten-free waffles

Gluten free • vegetarian • low carb • high protein • keto-friendly

MAKES: 16 rolls
PREP: 5 minutes
COOK: 10 minutes

Ingredients

3 eggs

1 tsp vanilla extract

½ cup milk

2 cups almond meal

1 tsp baking powder

melted butter, for greasing

Greek yoghurt, strawberries, maple syrup and toasted almonds to serve

Method

Switch on your waffle maker.

Whisk together the eggs, vanilla extract, milk, almond meal and baking powder to form a smooth batter.

Brush your waffle maker with melted butter then dollop about 2 tablespoons of batter onto the griddle and close the lid. Cook for around 5 minutes until waffle is crisp and puffy.

Serve with yoghurt, chopped strawberries, maple syrup and toasted almonds.

Tip

Want a vegan version? Sub the eggs with a banana and serve with soy or coconut yoghurt.

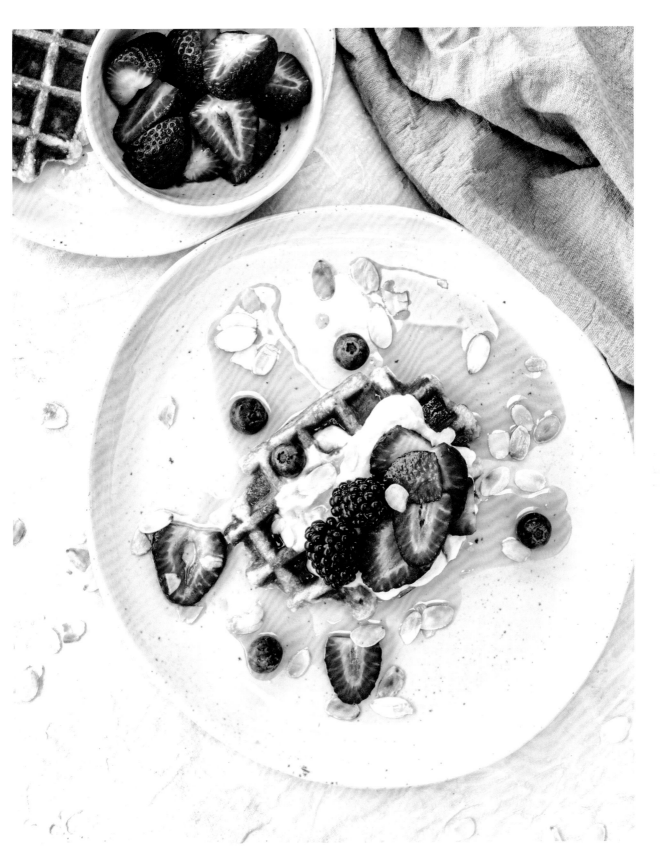

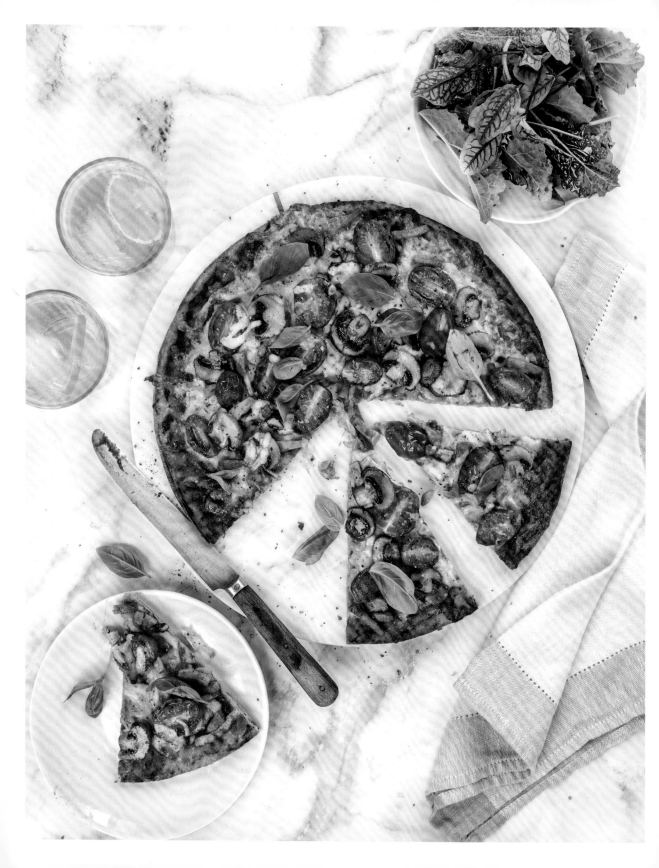

Low-carb breakfast pizza

Gluten free • vegetarian • low carb • keto-friendly

SERVES: 2
PREP: 5 minutes
COOK: 10 minutes

Ingredients

Pizza dough

1 cup grated mozzarella cheese

1 cup almond meal

2 tbsp cream cheese

1 egg, beaten

Topping

¼ cup passata

¼ cup mozzarella cheese

6 button mushrooms, sliced

6 cherry tomatoes, sliced

½ cup basil leaves

Method

Preheat the oven to 180°C.

Make the dough by placing the grated cheese, almond meal and cream cheese in a microwave-safe bowl and heating in the microwave for 1 minute. Remove from the microwave. Add the egg and stir vigorously until combined into a dough.

Sprinkle a little almond flour on your benchtop to avoid sticking. Roll out your pizza to the desired thickness.

Bake on a pizza tray in the oven for 10 minutes. Turn the base over and bake for a further 5 minutes.

Remove from the oven and top with the passata, cheese, mushrooms, and cherry tomatoes. Return pizza to the oven and bake until the cheese is melted and the mushrooms are cooked through.

Top with basil leaves and serve.

Tip

Want a vegan version? Use vegan mozzarella, vegan cream cheese and sub the egg for 1 tablespoon aquafaba (chickpea water).

Corn fritters

Vegetarian • high fibre

Ingredients

¼ cup Greek yoghurt

1 avocado mashed

½ lemon, squeezed

3 cups fresh corn kernels

3 long green shallots (spring onions), finely sliced

2 eggs, whisked

1 cup wholemeal flour

1 tsp baking powder

salt and pepper, to taste

2 tbsp olive oil

smoked salmon, rocket and lemon wedges, to serve

Method

Mix the yoghurt, avocado and lemon juice in a small bowl and set aside.

Mix the corn, spring onions, eggs, wholemeal flour, baking powder and seasoning to form the fritter batter.

Preheat the oven to 160°C.

Heat the olive oil in a frying pan over medium heat. Cook the fritters in batches, a few spoonfuls at a time. Cook for 2–3 minutes on each side.

Transfer to a baking tray and keep warm in the oven while you make the rest of the fritters.

Serve with avocado salsa, smoked salmon, rocket and lemon wedges.

Tip

Want a vegan version? Sub the egg for 2 tablespoons of aquafaba, use soy yoghurt and omit the salmon.

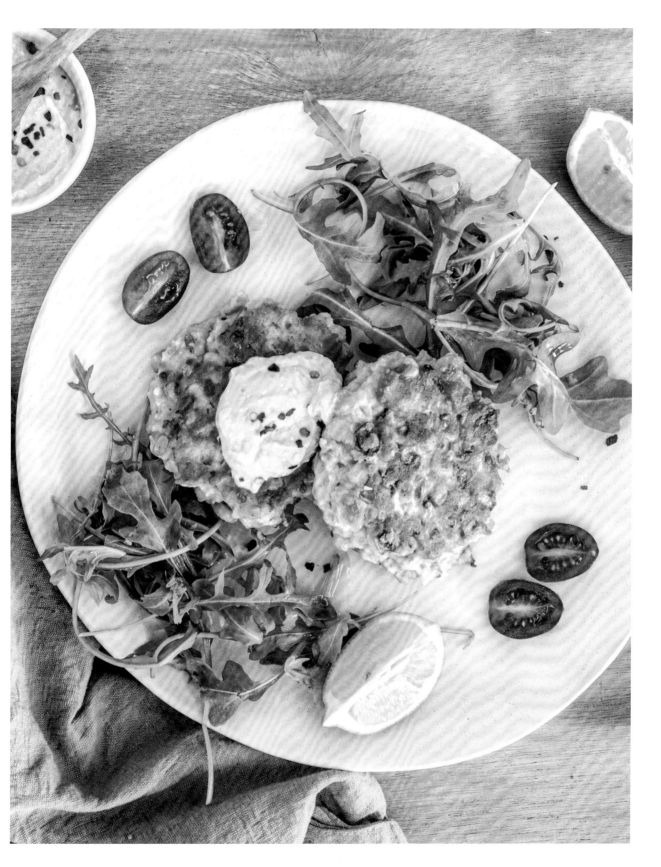

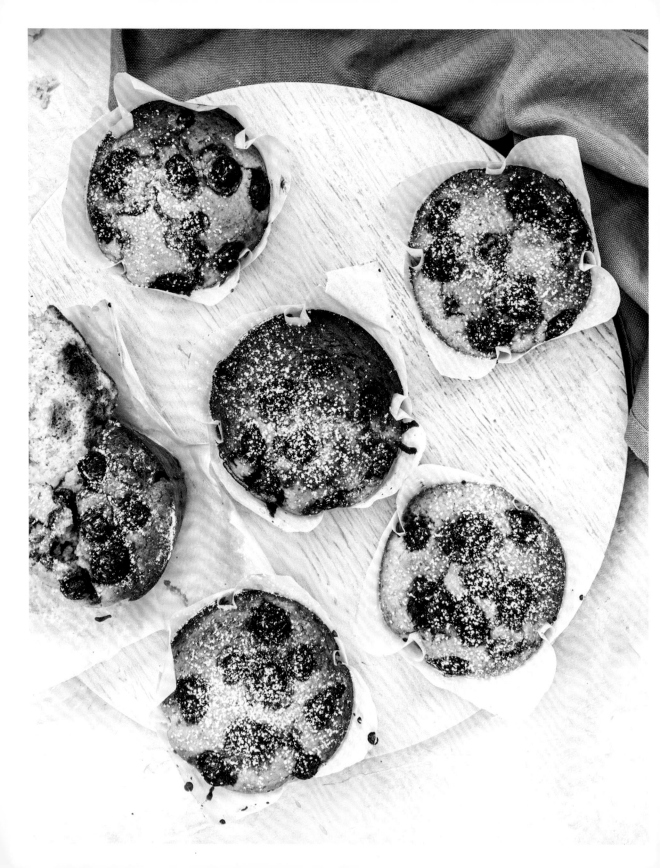

Blueberry breakfast muffins

Gluten free • vegetarian • gut-friendly • low carb • keto-friendly

MAKES: 12
PREP: 5 minutes
COOK: 25 minutes

Ingredients

300 g almond meal

2 tsp baking powder

60 g monkfruit sweetener

3 eggs

zest of 1 lemon

120 g kefir

50 g extra virgin olive oil

1 tsp vanilla extract

125 g blueberries

Method

Preheat the oven to 180°C. Line a muffin tray with muffin papers.

Place the dry ingredients in a bowl and lightly whisk until combined. Add the eggs, lemon zest, kefir, olive oil and vanilla extract and whisk until you get a smooth batter. Fold in the blueberries.

Divide batter evenly between muffin papers and bake for 20–25 minutes or until a skewer inserted into the centre comes out clean.

Transfer to a wire rack and let cool for 15 minutes before removing from muffin tray.

Tip
Want a vegan version? Sub the egg for 2 tablespoons of aquafaba and use soy yoghurt instead of kefir.

Orange teacake muffins

Gluten free • vegetarian • refined sugar free
• low carb • high protein • keto-friendly

MAKES: 12
PREP: *5 minutes*
COOK: *25 minutes*

Ingredients

1 Earl Grey tea bag

¼ cup of boiling water

⅓ cup oat milk

2 large eggs, whisked

1 tsp baking powder

⅔ cup monkfruit extract

2 cups almond meal

2 scoops vegan protein powder

1 tablespoon sugar free marmalade

1 cup monkfruit icing sugar

2 tablespoons fresh orange juice

Method

Preheat the oven to 180°C. Line a muffin tray with muffin papers.

Steep the teabag in the water for 5 minutes in a medium-sized bowl then remove the bag. Add the oat milk and eggs then fold in the dry ingredients.

Divide mix between muffin cases and cook for 15 minutes or until springy to touch.

Let cool and make the icing by mixing the icing sugar with the orange juice and marmalade. Spoon over muffins and serve.

Tip
Want a vegan version? Sub the egg for 2 tablespoons of aquafaba or 2 tablespoons apple sauce.

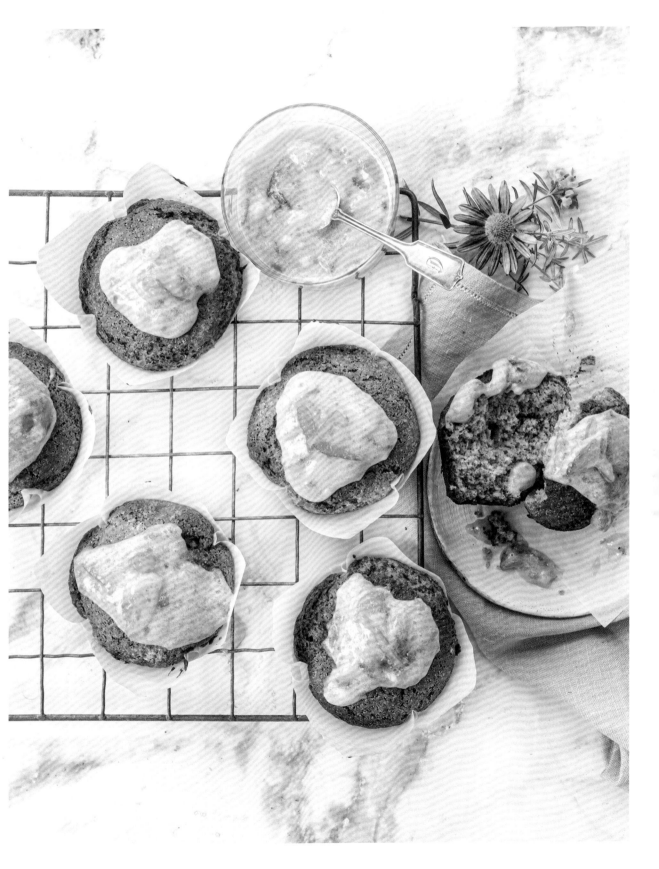

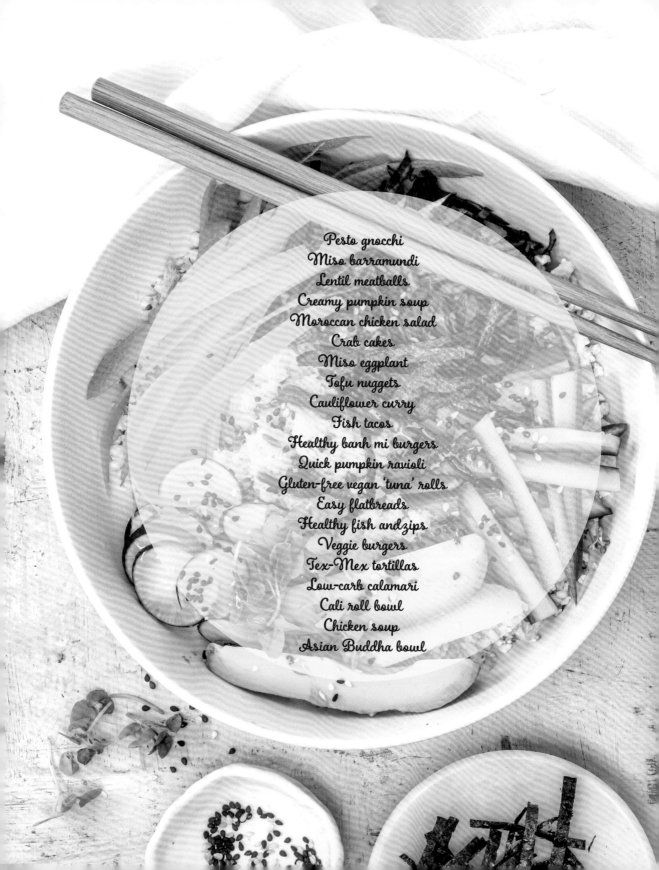

Pesto gnocchi
Miso barramundi
Lentil meatballs
Creamy pumpkin soup
Moroccan chicken salad
Crab cakes
Miso eggplant
Tofu nuggets
Cauliflower curry
Fish tacos
Healthy banh mi burgers
Quick pumpkin ravioli
Gluten-free vegan 'tuna' rolls
Easy flatbreads
Healthy fish and zips
Veggie burgers
Tex-Mex tortillas
Low-carb calamari
Cali roll bowl
Chicken soup
Asian Buddha bowl

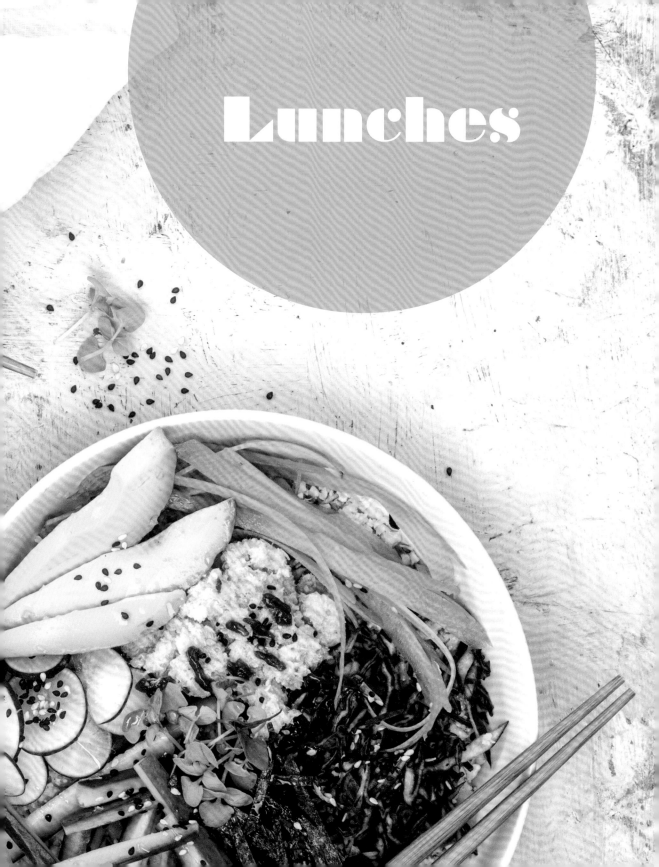

Lunches

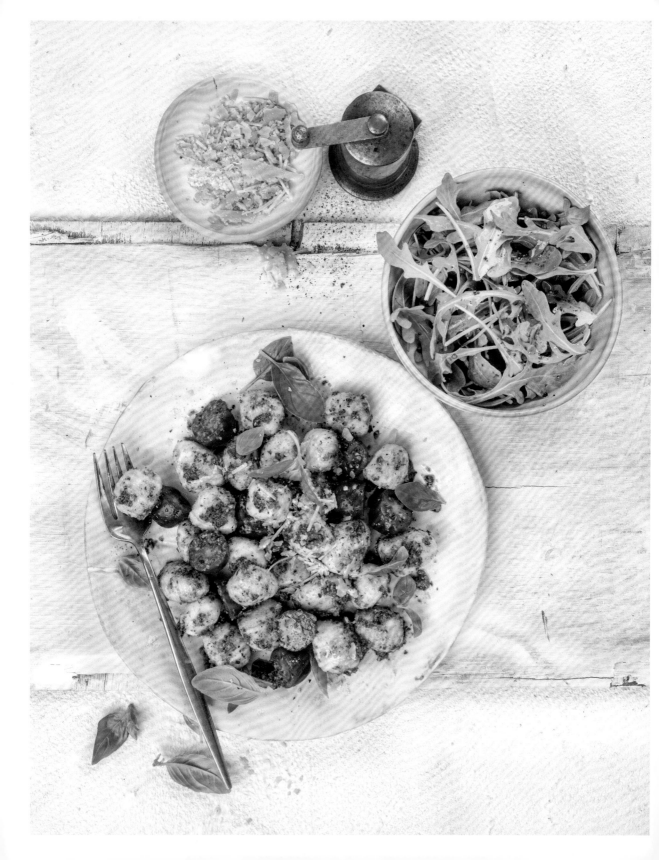

Pesto gnocchi

Gluten free • vegetarian • low carb • high protein
• high fibre • keto-friendly

SERVES: 4
PREP: 10 minutes
COOK: 25 minutes

Ingredients

Gnocchi

500 g cauliflower, steamed

¾ cup grated parmesan cheese

1 cup almond meal

2 egg yolks

1 tsp psyllium husk

1 cup shredded mozzarella cheese

2 tbsp olive oil

Pesto

½ cup olive oil

¾ cup grated parmesan cheese

3 tbsp walnuts

½ cup fresh basil

1 garlic clove

Method

Blend steamed cauliflower in a food processor until smooth. Transfer to a clean tea towel and squeeze out excess liquid. Return cauliflower to the food processor and add the parmesan cheese, almond meal, egg yolks and psyllium husk and blitz until smooth.

Melt cheese in microwave and add to the cauliflower mixture. Pulse until combined.

Shape mix into small balls (you should get around 12) and press each ball lightly with a fork. Refrigerate balls for 30 minutes.

Meanwhile, make the pesto by blending all the ingredients in a food processor until well combined.

Fry the gnocchi in olive oil until golden. Add the pesto and serve immediately.

Tip

This gnocchi recipe also works well with a simple sage butter.

Miso barramundi

Gluten free • low carb • high protein • keto-friendly

SERVES: 2
PREP: 10 minutes
COOK: 20 minutes

Ingredients

½ cup butter

3 tbsp red miso paste

¼ tsp smoked paprika

2 garlic cloves, crushed

1 lemon, juiced

1 tsp freshly chopped
    coriander

1 tbsp olive oil

2 barramundi fillets
    with skin on (125 g each)

Method

In a pan melt the butter, miso, paprika, garlic, lemon and coriander over low heat and set aside.

Heat the oil in a griddle pan on medium heat. Place the barramundi skin-side down and cook for 10–15 minutes until the skin is crispy and the flesh turns white.

Flip the fish over and add the sauce to the pan, being careful not to wet the crispy skin. Cook for 2–3 minutes and remove from the pan and place on a plate. Spoon sauce over and serve with a little fresh lemon.

Tip
Up your veggie and fibre intake and serve with spiralised zucchini and buckwheat noodles. Want a vegan version? Use pan-fried tempeh instead.

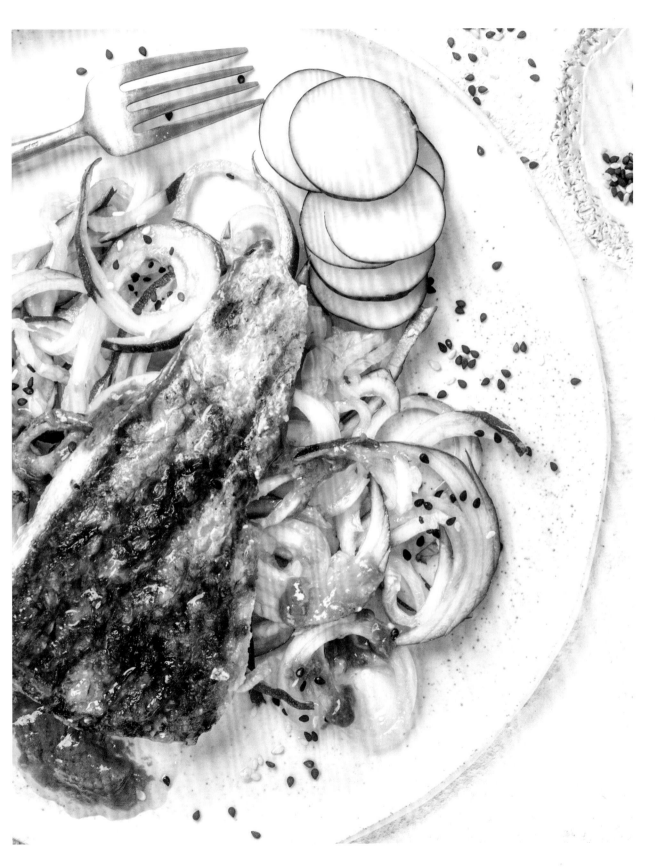

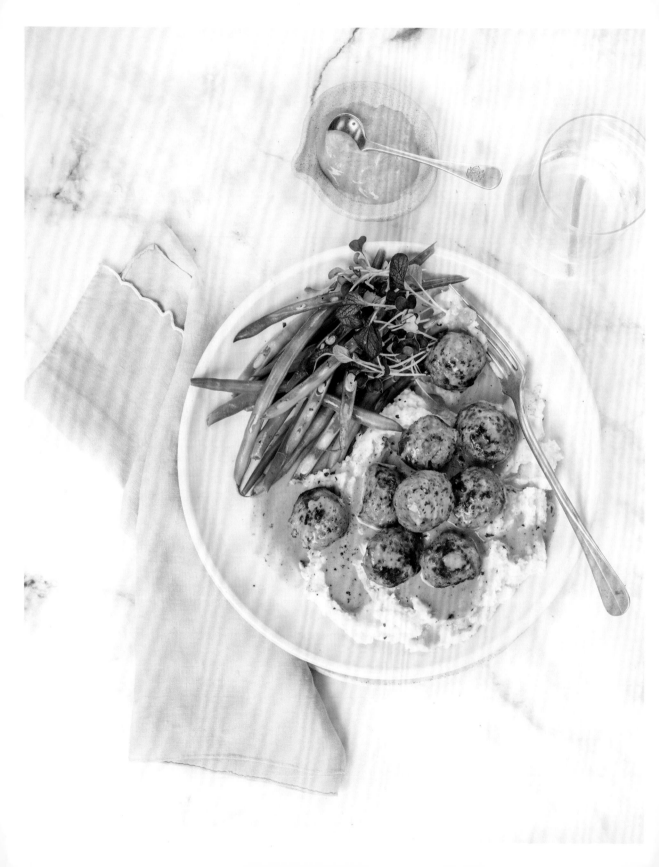

Lentil meatballs

Vegan • gut-friendly • high protein • high fibre

SERVES: 4
PREP: 10 minutes
COOK: 45 minutes

Ingredients

400 g tin brown lentils

1 onion, diced

6 garlic cloves, minced

1 cup sliced mushrooms

1 tsp ground cumin

¾ cup oats

1 tsp Dijon mustard

1 tsp dried Italian herbs

2 tbsp soy sauce

1 cup veggie stock

1 can coconut milk

1 tsp cornflour

Method

Preheat the oven to 180°C. Line a baking tray with baking paper.

Drain the lentils and set aside. Heat a little olive oil in a pan over medium heat and sauté the onion until translucent. Add the garlic, mushrooms and cumin and cook until softened.

Process the oats in a food processor until flour is formed. Add the lentils and veggies and blend until well combined.

Roll the veggie mix into small balls and place on the baking tray. Spray with olive oil and cook in the oven for about 25 minutes until golden.

Meanwhile, to make the sauce, put the Dijon mustard, herbs, soy sauce and coconut milk in a pan over low–medium heat. In a small bowl mix together the cornstarch with a little water and add to the gravy mixture. Whisk until you get your desired thickness.

Serve the meatballs with sauce and some mashed cauliflower and green beans.

Tip
You can make a healthy meat version using turkey mince instead of lentils.

Creamy pumpkin soup

Vegan • gut-friendly • high fibre

SERVES: 4
PREP: 10 minutes
COOK: 15 minutes

Ingredients

1 white onion, diced

400 g pumpkin, diced

6 garlic cloves, crushed

1 tsp ground cumin

1 tsp coriander

salt and pepper, to taste

1 can coconut milk

1 cup vegetable stock

coconut cream, to serve

Method

Heat a large saucepan over medium heat and sauté the onions, pumpkin and garlic in olive oil for 3–5 minutes until softened.

Add the cumin, coriander and salt and pepper to taste and cook for a further 2–5 minutes until fragrant.

Add the coconut milk and vegetable stock. Bring to the boil then reduce to a simmer and cook for a further 5–7 minutes until the veggies are tender.

Let cool for 5 minutes before blending until smooth.

Serve with a little coconut cream.

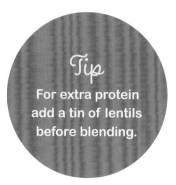

Tip
For extra protein add a tin of lentils before blending.

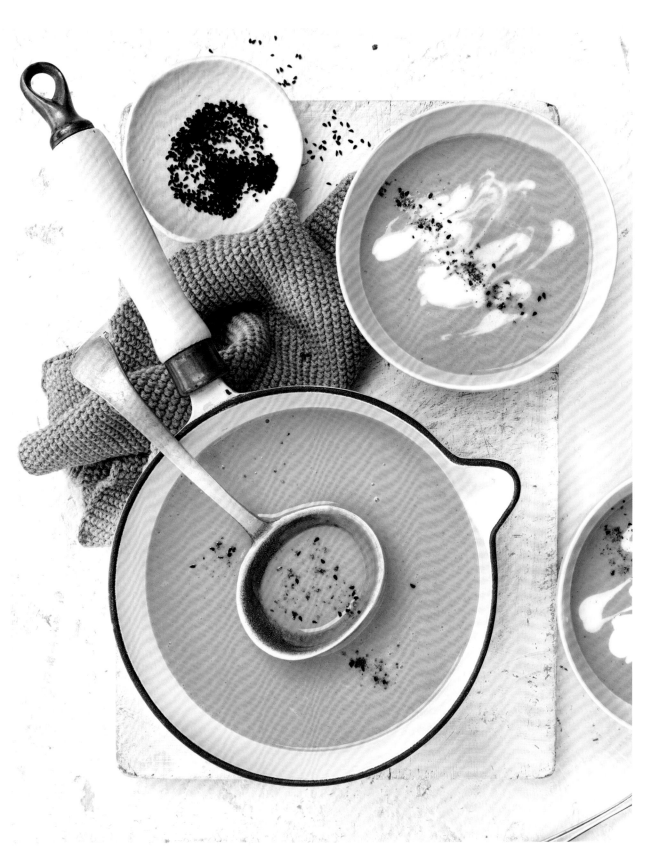

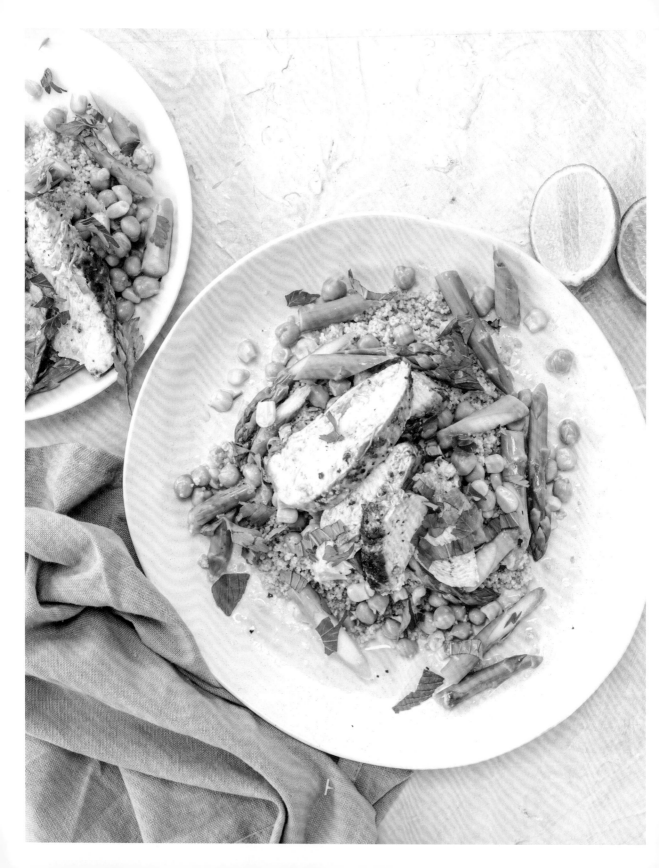

Moroccan chicken salad

Gut-friendly • high protein • high fibre

SERVES: 4
PREP: 10 minutes
COOK: 5 minutes

Ingredients

1 cup wholewheat couscous

500 g skinless chicken breast fillets, fat trimmed

2 tbsp Moroccan seasoning

300 g can sweetcorn, drained and rinsed

400 g can chickpeas, drained and rinsed

1 bunch asparagus, trimmed, cut into thirds, blanched

handful parsley leaves

handful mint leaves

2 tbsp olive oil

zest and juice of 1 lemon

1 tsp ground cumin

1 garlic clove, minced

60 g feta cheese, crumbled

Method

Cook cous cous according to packet instructions. Fluff with a fork and set aside.

Meanwhile, rub chicken with Moroccan seasoning. Pan fry chicken for 4 to 5 minutes each side over medium–high heat, or until cooked through. Set aside to rest for 5 minutes. Thickly slice chicken.

In a large bowl, combine couscous, corn, chickpeas, asparagus, parsley and mint.

In a jar, combine the olive oil, lemon juice and zest, cumin, and minced garlic. Shake well to combine.

Drizzle couscous salad mix with dressing and toss to coat. Top with chicken and sprinkle with feta to serve.

Tip

Want a vegan version? Sub the chicken for firm tofu and use vegan feta.

Crab cakes

Gluten free • low carb • high protein
• keto-friendly

SERVES: 4
PREP: 15 minutes
COOK: 10 minutes

Ingredients

1 egg

1 cup chopped fresh crab meat

1 tbsp mayonnaise

1 tbsp Dijon mustard

1 tbsp minced garlic

pinch of salt

¼ cup chopped fresh coriander

½ cup almond meal

2 tbsp olive oil

Method

Lightly whisk the egg in a medium bowl and mix in the crab meat, mayonnaise, mustard, garlic and salt until well combined. Fold in the coriander and almond meal.

Place tablespoons of mixture into a medium-size scone cutter and press down to form a pattie around 1 cm thick. You should be able to make about four patties. Refrigerate for 15 minutes.

Heat the oil in a frying pan over a medium heat. Fry the patties for around 5 minutes each side until golden brown.

Tip

Want a vegan version? Sub the crab meat and egg for a tin of chickpeas. Simply mash together with the liquid. Omit the mayo or use vegan mayo instead.

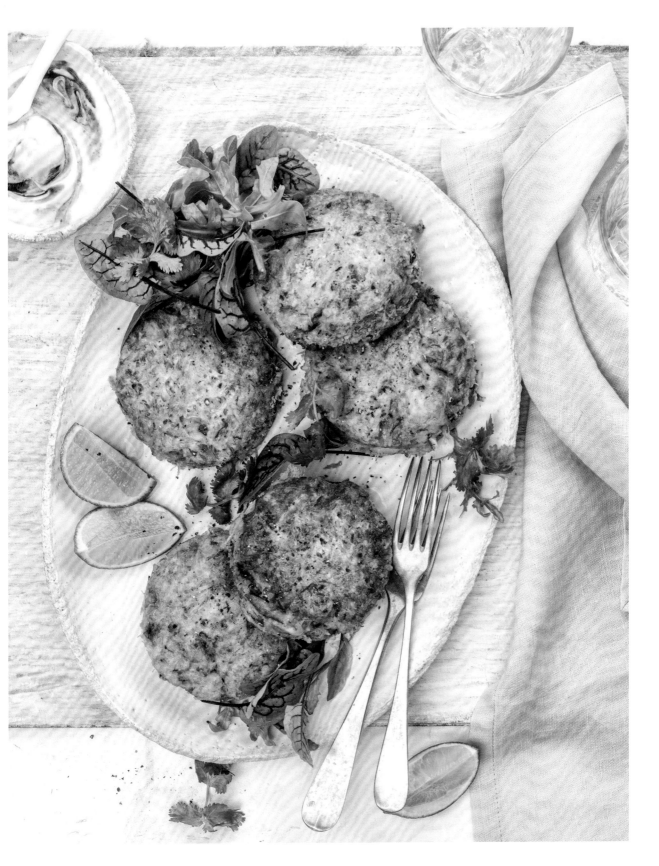

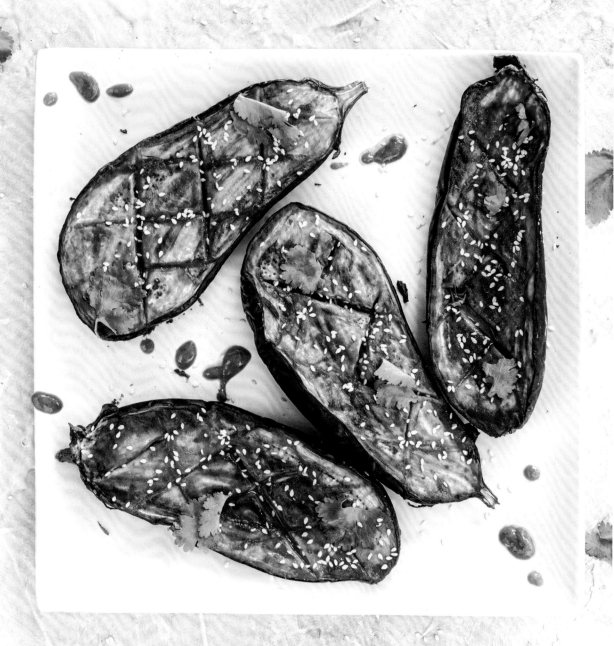

Miso eggplant

Vegan • gut-friendly • high fibre

SERVES: 4
PREP: 10 minutes
COOK: 15 minutes

Ingredients

4 small eggplants, halved
sea salt
¼ cup white miso paste
¼ cup mirin
1 tbsp coconut sugar
1 tbsp sesame oil
1 tbsp freshly minced ginger
1 tbsp sesame seeds
coriander leaves, to serve

Method

Preheat oven to 180°C.

Score eggplants in diamond shapes and pat dry. Rub with salt and set aside for 30 minutes on a baking tray. Pat the eggplants dry again using a paper towel and brush off the salt.

Place the miso paste, mirin, sugar, sesame oil and ginger in a small heavy bottomed saucepan on medium heat. Bring to a gentle boil, stirring constantly. Remove from heat.

Using a pastry brush, baste the eggplants with the miso sauce, reserving a little for later.

Bake the eggplants in the oven for 30 minutes until tender.

Remove from the oven, brush with the remaining glaze and top with sesame seeds and coriander leaves before serving.

Tip
Serve with brown rice and grilled salmon or tempeh for a nutritious and hearty lunch.

Tofu nuggets

Vegetarian • low carb • high fibre • keto-friendly

SERVES: 4
PREP: 10 minutes
COOK: 10 minutes

Ingredients

1 block firm tofu
1 tsp salt
1 tsp olive oil
¼ cup coconut flour
1 tsp smoked paprika
1 tsp garlic powder
½ tsp cracked black pepper
1 egg, whisked
olive oil spray

Method

Cut the tofu into 16 nugget-sized pieces and dry off on paper towel to reduce moisture.

In a bowl combine the tofu with the salt and olive oil.

In another bowl combine the coconut flour with the smoked paprika, garlic powder and cracked black pepper.

In a small bowl whisk the egg.

Dip each nugget in the egg and then coat in the coconut flour mixture. Set aside on a plate.

Heat a frying pan over a medium heat. Spray a little olive oil in the pan and fry the nuggets in batches for around 5 minutes each side, or if you have an air fryer cook on 180°C for 10 minutes.

Transfer the nuggets to a platter and serve.

Tip
Want a vegan version? Sub the egg for a tablespoon of aquafaba.

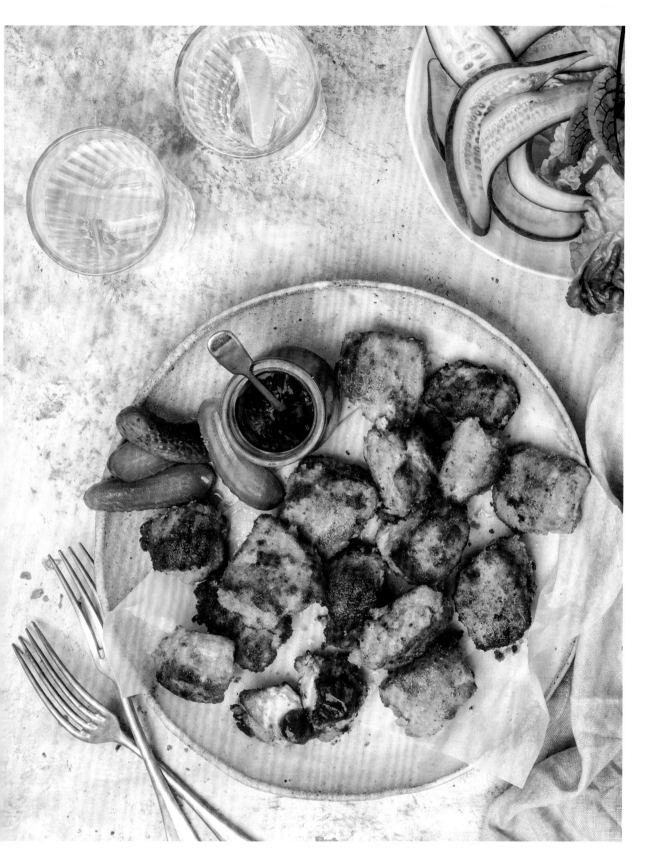

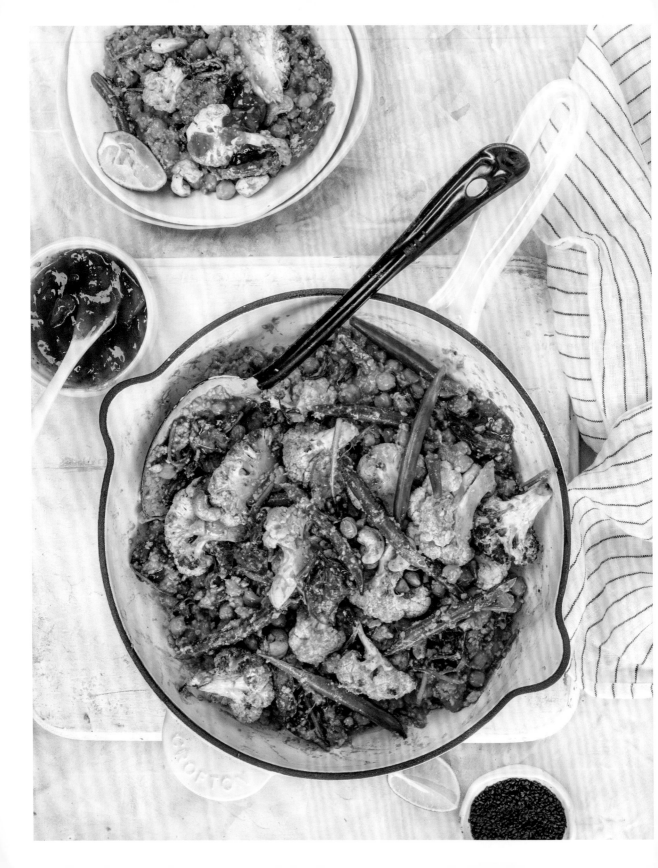

Cauliflower curry

Vegan • gut-friendly • high fibre

SERVES: 4
PREP: 10 minutes
COOK: 25 minutes

Ingredients

1 cauliflower

½ tsp garam masala

1 tbsp olive oil

1 cup raw cashews

¼ cup boiling water

2 cloves garlic

½ tsp ground turmeric

1 tsp black nigella seeds

1 tbsp tomato paste

400 g tin chickpeas,
    rinsed and drained

200 g green beans

200 g spinach leaves

handful of roasted cashews
    and coconut yoghurt, to
    serve

Method

Preheat oven to 220°C. Line a baking tray with baking paper.

Break the cauliflower into florets and place them in a large bowl with the garam masala and olive oil. Toss to coat. Place on the baking tray and cook for 20 minutes or until tender and lightly charred.

While the cauliflower is roasting, make the curry paste by placing the cashews and boiling water in a small bowl to soak for 5 minutes.

Place the garlic, turmeric, black mustard seeds and tomato paste in a food processor and process until finely chopped. Drain the cashews, add to the processor and process until smooth.

Heat a little oil in a large heavy-based frying pan over medium heat. Add the curry paste and cook, stirring, for 3 minutes. Add a quarter of a cup of water and bring to a simmer.

Add the chickpeas and beans and cook for 4–6 minutes or until tender. Roughly chop the roasted cashews.

Stir the cauliflower through the curry and serve with spinach leaves, yoghurt and a sprinkle of cashews.

Tip

Serve with brown rice or quinoa to up the fibre. If you're not following a vegetarian or vegan diet you can add some firm white fish such as basa to up the protein and omega-3s.

Fish tacos

Gluten free • low carb • high protein • high fibre
• keto-friendly

SERVES: 4
PREP: 10 minutes
COOK: 10 minutes

Ingredients

2 basa fillets
1 tbsp olive oil
2 tbsp dukkah seasoning
4 red cabbage leaves
½ carrot, julienned
½ cucumber, julienned
1 tbsp tahini
1 lemon wedge

Method

Preheat a BBQ grill or chargrill pan over medium heat.

Rub both sides of the basa fillets with the oil and dukkah. Grill for about 2–3 minutes on each side. Remove from the grill and slice into pieces.

Fill the cabbage leaves with the fish, carrot and cucumber and drizzle with tahini and a squeeze of lemon.

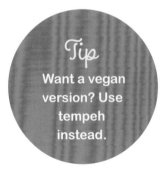

Tip
Want a vegan version? Use tempeh instead.

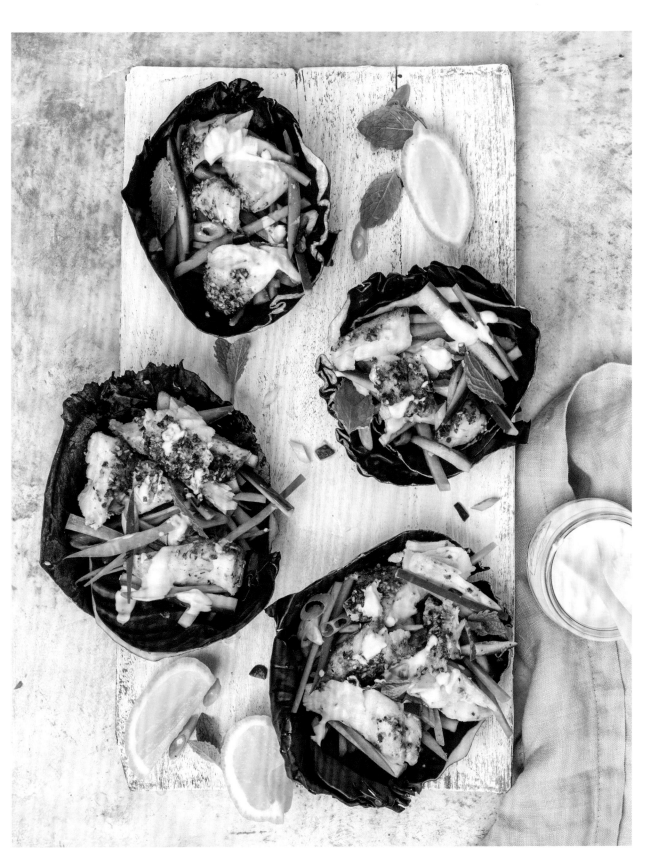

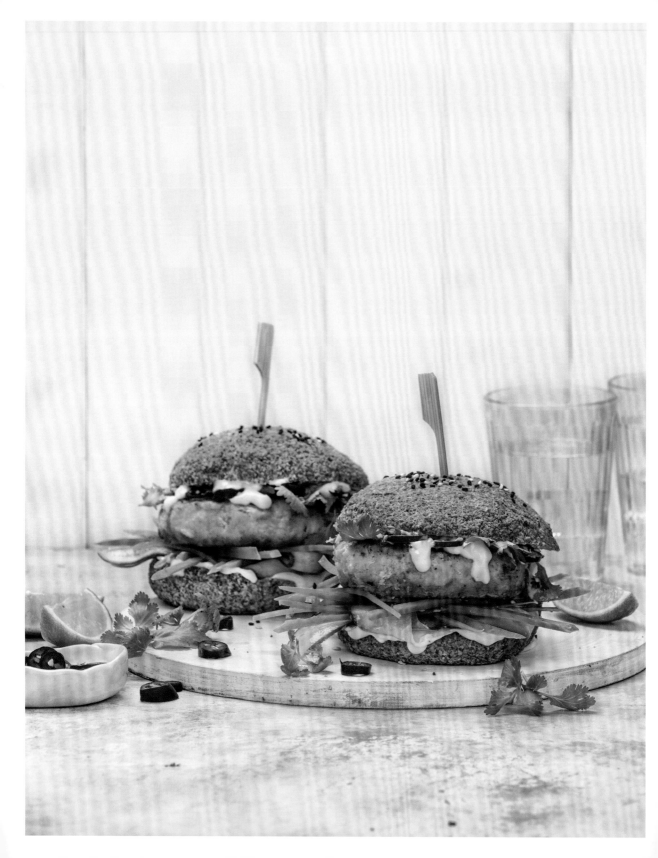

Healthy banh mi burgers

Gluten free • low carb • high protein • high fibre • keto-friendly

Ingredients

The buns

1 cup almond meal

2 tbsp psyllium husk

1 tsp bicarb (baking) soda

1 tbsp apple cider vinegar

½ cup boiling water

2 egg whites

sesame seeds

The burgers

225 g chicken mince

½ long green shallot (spring onion), finely chopped

½ tsp freshly grated ginger

½ tsp freshly minced garlic

1 tsp tamari sauce

juice of ½ a lime

2 tbsp mayo

½ carrot, julienned

1 cucumber thinly sliced in strips

coriander leaves to serve

freshly sliced red chilli (optional)

Method

Preheat the oven to 180°C. Line a baking sheet with baking paper.

Combine the almond flour with the psyllium husk and bicarb soda in a medium bowl. Add the apple cider vinegar, boiling water and egg whites and mix to form a gooey dough. Split the dough into two pieces, roll into bread rolls and top with sesame seeds. Place on a baking sheet and bake for 30 minutes until golden brown, the bottom is crisp and the bread roll sounds hollow when tapped.

Meanwhile, make the banh mi burgers by mixing the chicken mince with the spring onion, ginger, garlic, tamari and lime juice. Shape into two patties and fry in a pan over medium heat for 5 minutes each side, until golden brown and cooked through.

Slice the bread rolls and spread mayo on both halves. Top with cucumber, carrot, coriander, chilli, if desired, and the banh mi patties, and serve.

Tip
Want a vegan version? Use soy plant-based mince instead of chicken mince.

Quick pumpkin ravioli

Gut-friendly • high fibre

SERVES: 4
PREP: 15 minutes
COOK: 15 minutes

Ingredients

85 g pumpkin, peeled and diced into small cubes

1 clove garlic

1 tbsp olive oil

pinch of salt and freshly ground pepper

1 tbsp butter

2 tbsp ricotta

2 fresh lasagna sheets

100 g butter

1 clove garlic, minced

6 fresh sage leaves

prosciutto strips

grated parmesan, to serve

rocket, to serve

Method

Preheat the oven to 250°C. Line a baking tray with baking paper.

Toss the pumpkin on the tray with the whole garlic clove, olive oil and salt and pepper and roast for about 10 minutes until tender and soft.

Put the pumpkin and garlic in a food processor, add the butter and ricotta and pulse for a few minutes until well combined. Transfer the filling to a bowl and set aside.

Place the lasagna sheet on a flat surface and dollop the filling equally in 12 spots. I usually divide it three across and four down. Place the other lasagna sheet on top and use a small cookie cutter to cut out 12 circles of ravioli. Press down the edges to make sure the filling won't seep out.

Bring a pot of water to the boil and gently cook the ravioli for 3–5 minutes until tender. Drain and set aside.

Melt the butter in a pan over medium heat for a few minutes until golden, add the sage, prosciutto and then the ravioli. Fry for a few minutes before serving topped with parmesan cheese and some rocket.

Tip

Want a vegan version? Omit the prosciutto and use vegan ricotta and parmesan instead.

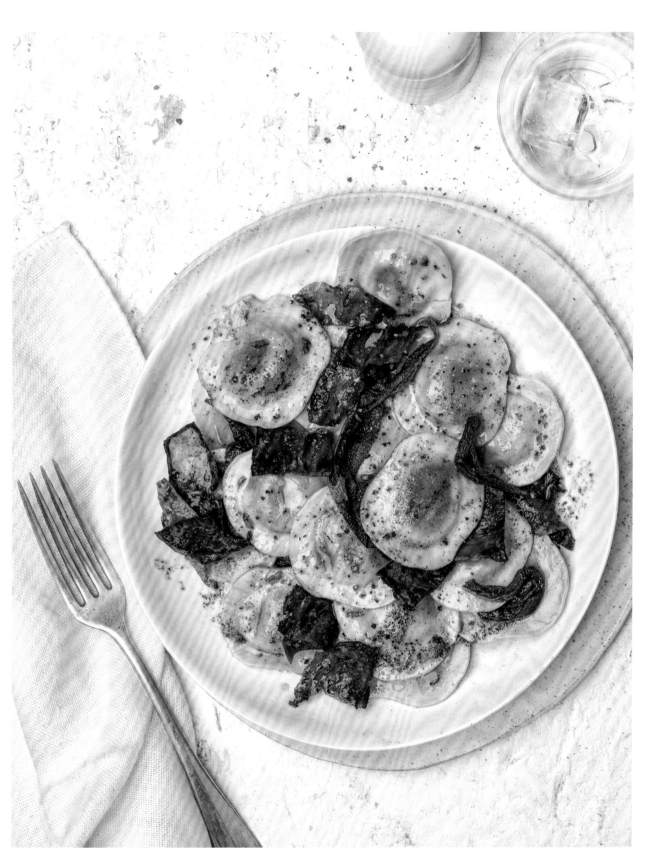

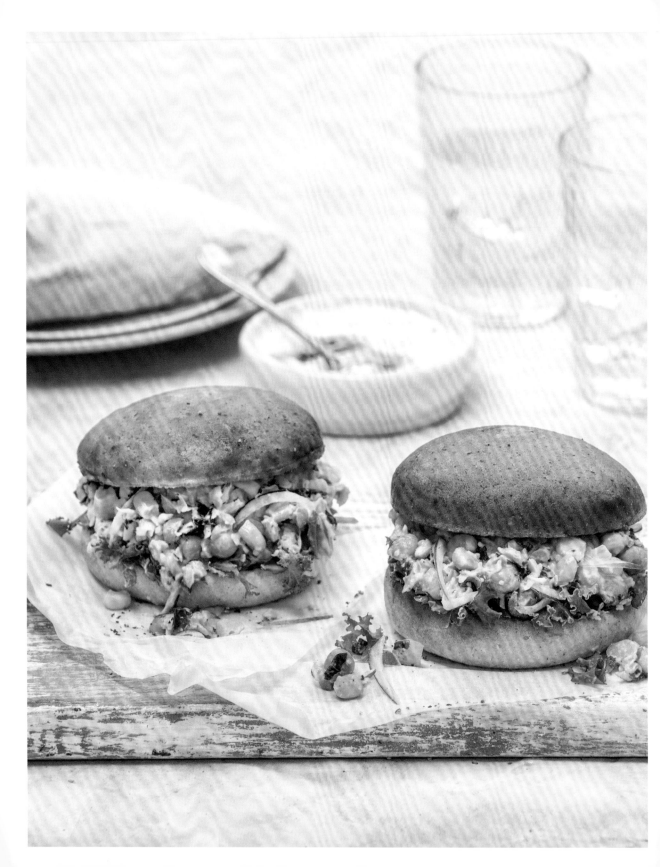

Gluten-free vegan 'tuna' rolls

Gluten free • vegan • gut-friendly • high fibre

SERVES: 2
PREP: 10 minutes

Ingredients

2 cups chickpeas

2 nori sheets

2 tbsp vegan mayo

2 tbsp lemon juice

1 cup sweetcorn, drained

1 small onion, finely diced

salt and pepper to taste

2 gluten-free sourdough buns, toasted

grated carrot and mixed leaves to serve

Method

Place the chickpeas in a bowl and mash with a fork, leaving some bigger bits for more texture.

Blend the nori sheet in a high-speed blender until you get nori flakes. Add the nori to the chickpeas. Add the rest of the ingredients and stir until well combined.

Spread a thick layer of the chickpea mix on your toasted bun and top with the grated carrot and mixed leaves.

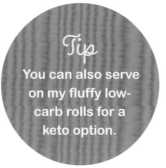

Tip
You can also serve on my fluffy low-carb rolls for a keto option.

Easy flatbreads

Gluten free • low carb • high protein • high fibre • keto-friendly

SERVES: 4
PREP: 15 minutes
COOK: 10 minutes

Ingredients

1½ tbsp psyllium husk

⅓ cup coconut flour

½ cup lukewarm water

1 tsp olive oil

½ tsp bicarb (baking) soda

½ tsp salt

1 tbsp olive oil

2 garlic cloves, minced

1 brown onion, diced

1 tsp ground cumin

1 tsp ground cinnamon

1 tsp smoked paprika

250 g turkey mince

2 ripe tomatoes, diced

Method

First make the flatbreads by mixing the psyllium husk and coconut flour in a bowl. Add the water, olive oil and bicarb soda and mix to create a dough. Knead the dough with your hands for one minute. If it is sticky, add a little extra coconut flour. Set the dough aside to rest for 10 minutes.

Meanwhile, make the topping by heating the olive oil in a frying pan over medium heat. Add the garlic and onion and sauté for 2–3 minutes until translucent. Add the cumin, cinnamon and paprika and fry for about a minute until fragrant.

Add the turkey and cook for a further 8 minutes or so until the meat is browned and cooked through.

Stir through the tomatoes and cook for another 5 minutes until cooked through.

Meanwhile, divide the dough into four equal balls. Roll the balls between two sheets of baking paper to around 20 centimetres in diameter. Heat a large frying pan over a medium heat and cook each flatbread for 2–3 minutes each side. Top with the turkey and serve.

Tip

Want a vegan version? Use soy plant-based mince instead of turkey mince.

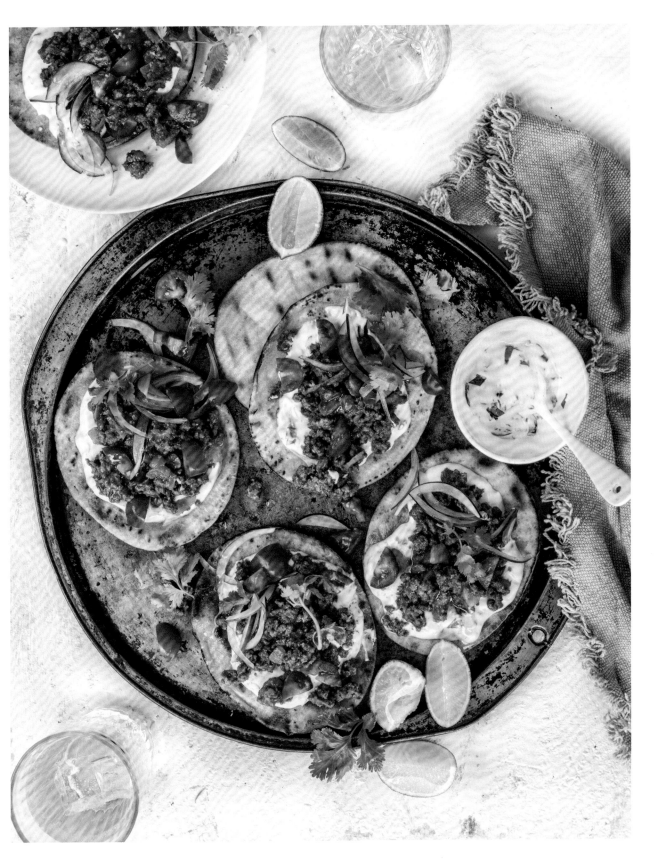

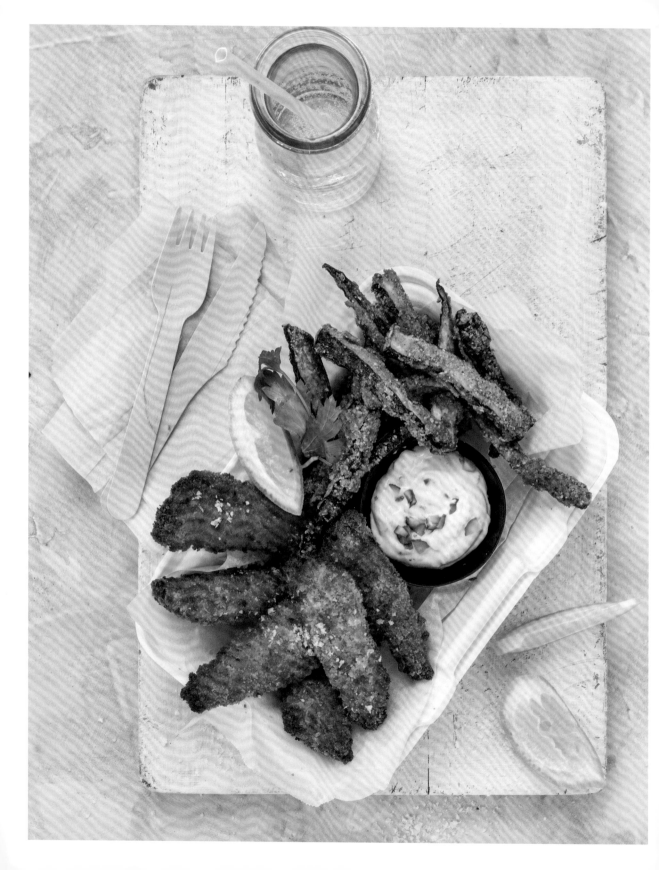

Healthy fish and zips

High protein • high fibre

SERVES: *2*
PREP: *5 minutes*
COOK: *15 minutes*

Ingredients

1 egg, whisked

½ cup wholewheat flour

½ tsp smoked paprika

½ tsp garlic powder

salt and pepper, to taste

225g cod (or other firm white fish), cut into pieces

1 zucchini cut into sticks

Method

Preheat the oven to 200°C. Line a baking sheet with baking paper.

Whisk the egg in a small bowl. In another bowl mix the flour, smoked paprika, garlic powder and seasoning.

Pat the fish dry with a paper towel before dipping in the egg and then the flour mixture. Repeat with the zucchini.

Place the battered fish and zucchini on the baking tray and bake in the oven for 15 minutes until crispy. You can also cook in the air fryer.

Tip

Want a vegan version? Replace the cod with oyster mushrooms soaked in vegan fish sauce. You can also use tofu.

Veggie burgers

Vegetarian • gut-friendly • high fibre

SERVES: 4
PREP: 5 minutes
COOK: 15 minutes

Ingredients

400 g plant-based soy mince

½ tsp ground cumin

½ tsp smoked paprika

¼ tsp cinnamon

salt and pepper, to taste

1 egg, whisked

½ cup wholemeal
    breadcrumbs

1 tbsp olive oil

75 g Greek goat's feta
    cheese

¼ cup cucumber, grated

¼ cup fresh mint

4 gluten-free sourdough
    buns, toasted

4 lettuce leaves

1 tomato, sliced

Method

Mix the soy mince with the cumin, smoked paprika, cinnamon, salt and pepper. Add the egg and breadcrumbs and mix thoroughly. Form the mince into two patties and set aside.

Heat the olive oil in a frying pan over medium heat and fry the patties for 5 minutes on each side.

In a food processor pulse together the goat's cheese, cucumber and mint until well blended.

Toast the buns lightly and spread the feta mixture on each bun. Top with the lettuce, tomato and patties and place the other bun half on top.

Tip

Want a vegan version? Replace the goat's feta with vegan feta and the egg with 1 tablespoon of aquafaba.

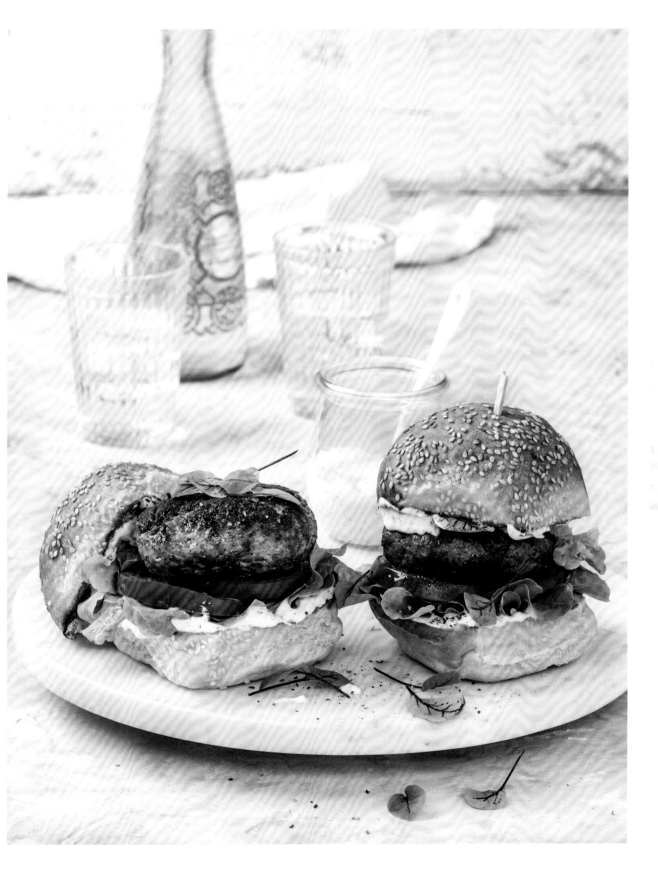

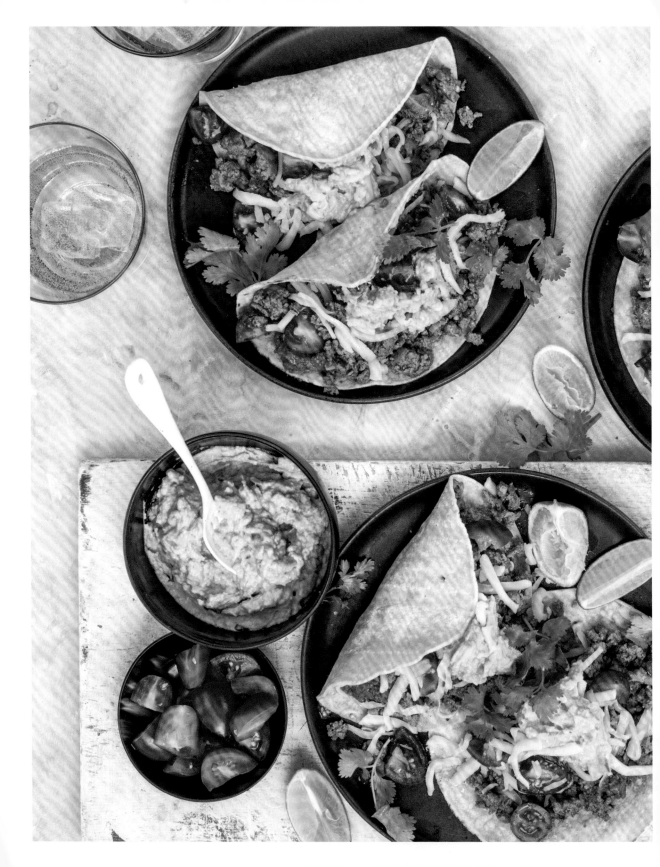

Tex-Mex tortillas

Vegetarian • high fibre • low carb • high protein

SERVES: 4
PREP: 5 minutes
COOK: 15 minutes

Ingredients

2 eggs

5 tbsp cream cheese

1 tbsp psyllium husk

1 tbsp coconut flour

1 tbsp olive oil

250 g plant-based soy mince

1 tbsp Mexican spice

salt and pepper to season

¼ cup water

¾ cup grated cheddar cheese

mashed avocado, lime and cherry tomatoes to serve

Method

Place the eggs and cream cheese in a bowl and beat with a hand mixer until smooth and fluffy. Fold in the psyllium husk and coconut flour until you have a smooth batter. Let sit for a minute or so until the batter thickens.

Heat a griddle pan over medium heat and add 2 tablespoons of batter for each tortilla. You should be able to make two for each person. Cook for 2–3 minutes each side until golden. Remove from the pan and set aside.

Heat a frying pan over medium heat and add the oil, soy mince, Mexican spice, salt and pepper and water and simmer for about 8–10 minutes until the liquid is absorbed and mince is cooked through.

Divide the mince between the tortillas, top with grated cheese, a dollop of mashed avocado, a squeeze of lime and some chopped cherry tomatoes.

Tip
Want a vegan version? Sub the cream and cheddar cheese for vegan options and the eggs for 2 tablespoons of aquafaba.

Low-carb calamari

Gluten free • low carb • high protein • high fibre • keto-friendly

SERVES: 4
PREP: 5 minutes
COOK: 5 minutes

Ingredients

⅓ cup vegan protein powder

1 tbsp coconut flour

1 tsp salt

1 tsp ground black pepper

300 g cleaned calamari tubes

olive oil

lemon wedges garlic mayo
   and rocket to serve

Method

Whisk together the protein powder, coconut flour and salt and pepper in a medium-size bowl.

Cut the calamari into 1-cm-thick rings and pat dry with a paper towel. Lightly toss the rings in the flour mix and dust off any excess mixture .

Heat a frying pan over a high heat, add some oil and fry in batches for about 2–4 minutes until the calamari is golden brown.

Serve immediately with lemon wedges, garlic mayo and a healthy serving of rocket.

Tip

Want a vegan version? Simply cut some king oyster mushrooms into rings and add powdered nori sheets into the flour mixture. Sub the mayo for vegan mayo, which can easily be made with aquafaba instead of eggs.

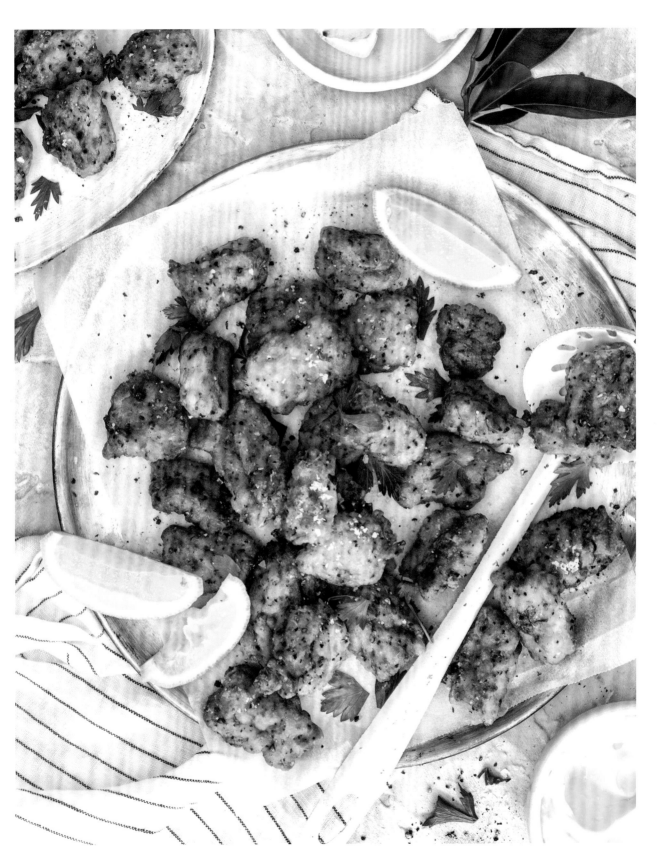

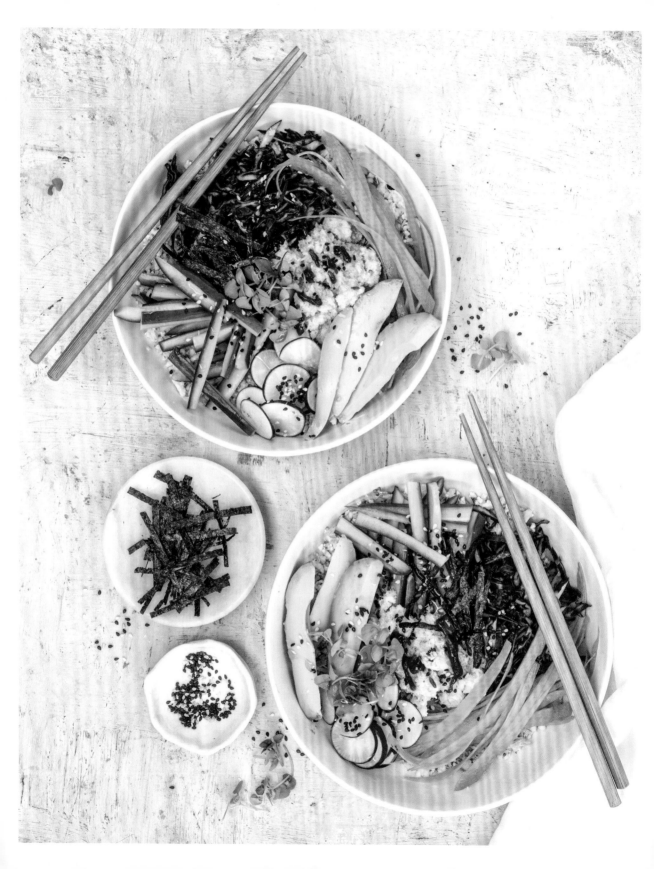

Cali roll bowl

Gluten free • gut-friendly • high protein • high fibre

SERVES: 4

PREP: 20 minutes

Ingredients

3 tbsp mayonnaise

1 tbsp water

2 tsp wasabi paste

400 g fresh crab meat

2 cups cooked brown rice

1 tbsp coconut oil, melted

1 tbsp sesame oil

1 tsp tamari sauce

1 avocado, sliced

1 nori sheet, cut into thin strips

1 Lebanese cucumber, sliced or in matchsticks

⅓ cup shredded red cabbage

1 radish, thinly sliced

1 small carrot, julienned

1 tsp sesame seeds

Method

Combine the mayonnaise, water and wasabi paste in a bowl and add the crab meat.

Add the coconut oil, sesame oil and tamari sauce to the rice and mix well. Divide the rice evenly between the bowls – around half a cup per person.

Top each serve with a quarter of the crab mixture, avocado slices, nori strips, cucumber, shredded cabbage, radish slices, and carrots. Sprinkle with sesame seeds.

Tip

Want a keto-friendly low-carb version? Sub the brown rice for riced cauliflower. Not keen on crab? Use tinned/ fresh salmon or tuna instead.

Chicken soup

Gluten free • low carb • high protein
• keto-friendly

SERVES: 4
PREP: 20 minutes
COOK: 1-2 hours

Ingredients

3 skinless chicken marylands
2 litres water
1 onion, peeled
1 carrot
2 sticks celery
1 bulb garlic, peeled
1 cup coconut cream
pumpkin seeds, to serve

Method

Place the chicken and water in a large pot over a medium heat. Add the onion, carrot, celery and garlic. Bring to the boil and simmer for at least 1 hour.

Remove the chicken from the pot and take the meat off the bones. Return the chicken meat to the pot, leaving a little aside for serving.

Let the soup cool for a few minutes. Add the coconut cream and blitz in a food processor or with a stick blender until thick and creamy.

Serve in bowls with the remaining chicken and some pumpkin seeds on top.

Tip

Want a vegan version? Use vegan chicken and vegan stock instead.

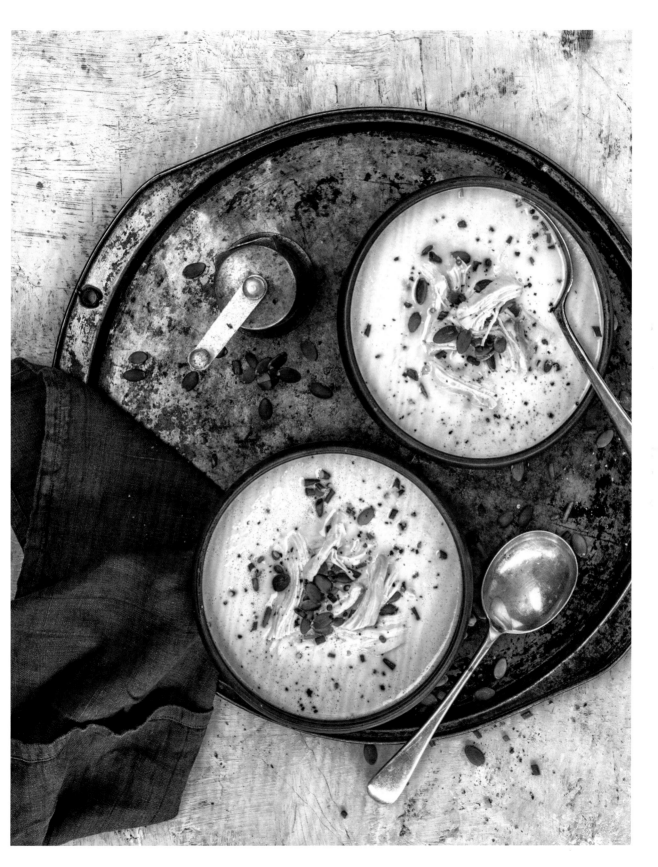

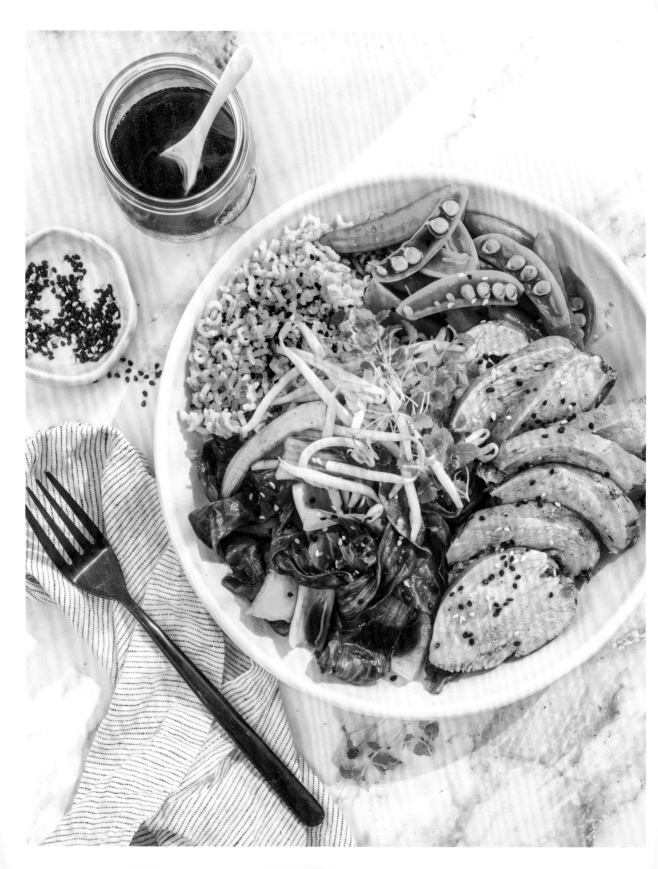

Asian Buddha bowl

Gluten free • gut-friendly • high protein • high fibre

SERVES: 2
PREP: 10 minutes
COOK: 15 minutes

Ingredients

1 cup water

1 whole star anise

1 Ceylon tea bag

1 tbsp coconut sugar

2 chicken breast fillets, trimmed

1 tbsp tamari sauce

2 tsp sesame oil

1 cup cooked brown rice

1 bunch bok choy, chopped and blanched

a handful of sugar snap peas, trimmed, blanched and halved

toasted sesame seeds and beansprouts, to serve

Method

Put the water, star anise, tea bag and sugar in a saucepan and bring to the boil. Add the chicken, reduce heat to a simmer and poach for about 15 minutes.

Remove the chicken and star anise and set the chicken aside for 10 minutes to rest. Reserve the liquid and add the sesame oil and tamari sauce.

Slice the chicken and arrange on the rice alongside the blanched veggies.

Drizzle with sauce and top with a sprinkle of sesame seeds and a few beansprouts.

Tip

Want a keto-friendly low-carb version? Sub the brown rice for riced cauliflower.

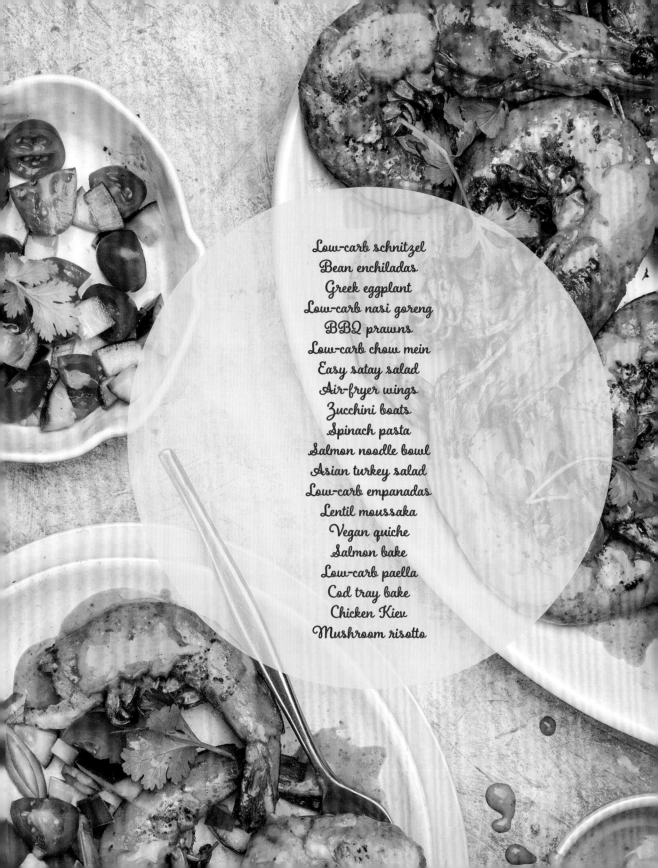

Low-carb schnitzel
Bean enchiladas
Greek eggplant
Low-carb nasi goreng
BBQ prawns
Low-carb chow mein
Easy satay salad
Air-fryer wings
Zucchini boats
Spinach pasta
Salmon noodle bowl
Asian turkey salad
Low-carb empanadas
Lentil moussaka
Vegan quiche
Salmon bake
Low-carb paella
Cod tray bake
Chicken Kiev
Mushroom risotto

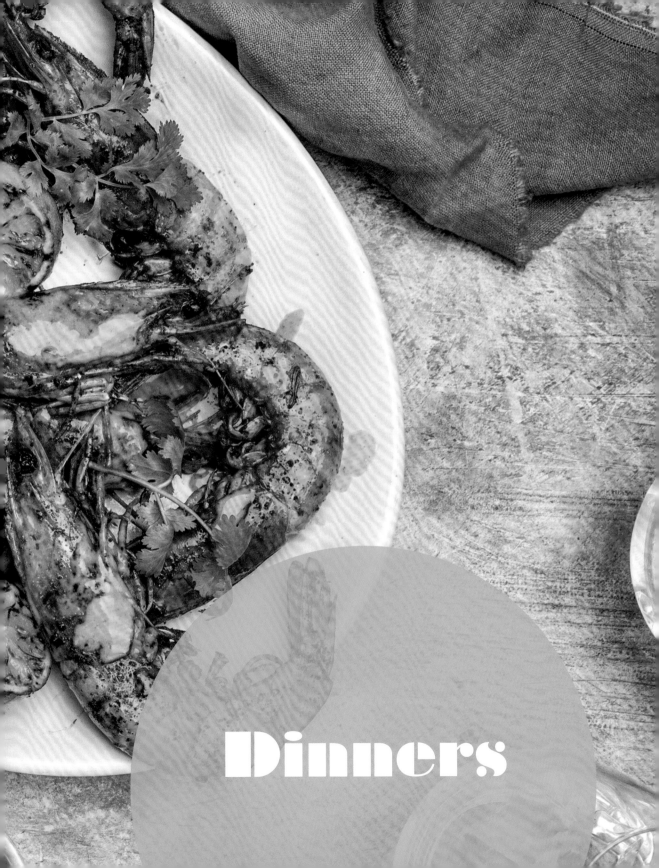

Dinners

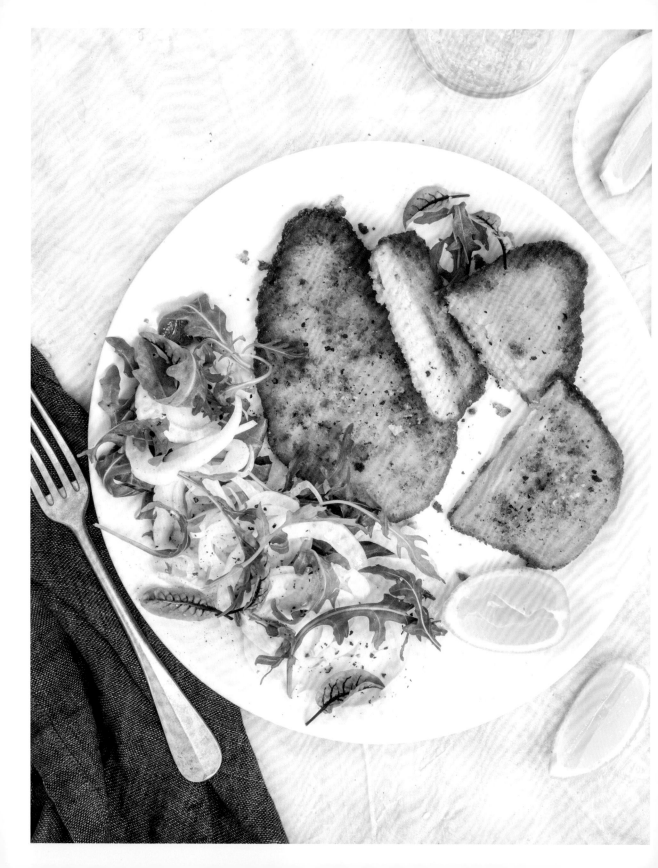

Low-carb schnitzel

Gluten free • low carb • high protein
• keto-friendly

SERVES: 4
PREP: 5 minutes
COOK: 15 minutes

Ingredients

¼ cup almond meal

¼ cup parmesan cheese, grated

¼ tsp lemon zest

¼ tsp paprika

¼ tsp salt

1 egg, beaten

2 skinless chicken breasts

1 tbsp olive oil

leafy greens and shaved fennel, to serve

Method

Mix the almond meal, parmesan, lemon zest, paprika and salt together in a bowl.

In another bowl, lightly beat the egg.

Cover the chicken with plastic wrap and pound it until flattened to around 5-mm thick.

Dip the chicken in the egg, then the almond meal mixture.

Heat the oil in a large frying pan. Once hot, fry the schnitzels for 5–8 minutes on each side, until golden brown and cooked through.

Serve with leafy greens and shaved fennel.

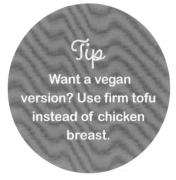

Tip
Want a vegan version? Use firm tofu instead of chicken breast.

Bean enchiladas

Vegetarian • low carb • high protein • high fibre

SERVES: 4
PREP: 5 minutes
COOK: 20 minutes

Ingredients

2 tbsp olive oil

1 onion, diced

400 g tin black beans, drained and rinsed

1 tsp ground cumin

½ tsp smoky paprika

salt and pepper, to taste

⅓ cup water

1 cup passata

2 tbsp sour cream

2 green chillies, chopped

4 low-carb wholewheat wraps

1 cup grated cheddar cheese

Method

Preheat oven to 220°C.

Heat the oil in a pan over medium heat and sauté the onion for 3–4 minutes or until the onion is translucent.

Add the beans and cook for about 3 minutes then add the cumin and smoked paprika and stir until fragrant. Add the salt and pepper to taste. Add the water and cook for about another 5 minutes.

Divide the mixture between the wraps and roll up and place lengthwise in a baking dish.

In a bowl mix the passata together with the sour cream and green chillies then drizzle over the wraps. Top with the cheese and bake for 15 minutes, until the cheese is melted and bubbling.

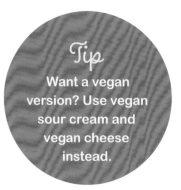

Tip
Want a vegan version? Use vegan sour cream and vegan cheese instead.

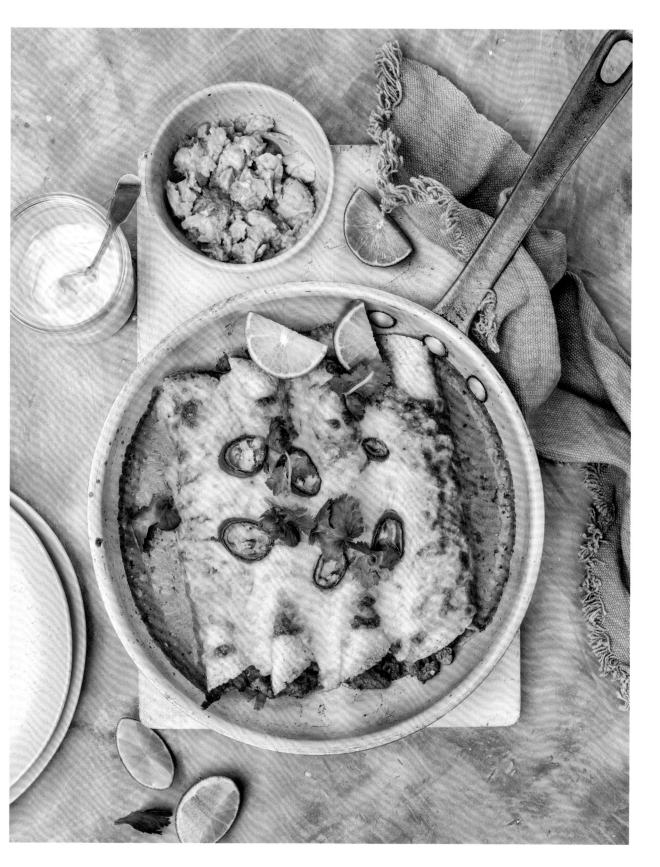

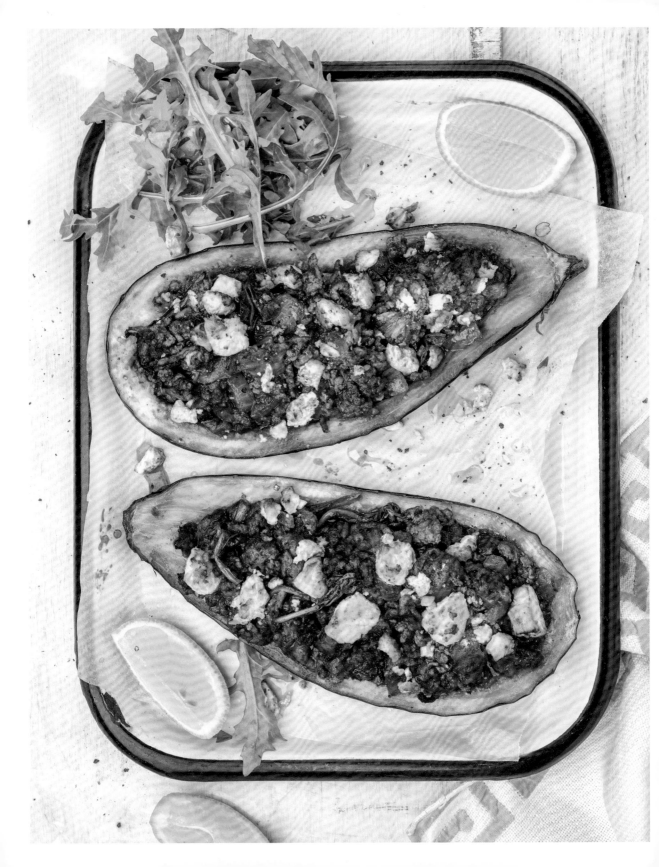

Greek eggplant

Vegetarian • low carb • high protein • high fibre

SERVES: 2
PREP: 5 minutes
COOK: 20 minutes

Ingredients

1 eggplant
1 tbsp olive oil
1 small onion, diced
3 garlic cloves, crushed
250 g plant-based soy mince
salt and pepper, to taste
pinch of cinnamon
pinch of smoky paprika
¼ cup passata
handful of baby spinach
½ cup Greek goat's feta,
    crumbled

Method

Preheat the oven to 200°C. Line a baking tray with baking paper.

Slice the eggplant lengthwise, scoop out the flesh, dice and set aside. Place eggplant shells on the baking tray.

Heat the oil in a pan over medium heat and sauté the onion and garlic for 3–4 minutes, or until the onion is translucent. Add the mince and cook for 4–5 minutes until browned. Add the salt and pepper, cinnamon, paprika and the diced eggplant flesh and cook for 5 minutes. Add the passata and simmer for 5 minutes. Stir through the spinach and allow to wilt.

Spoon the mince mixture into the eggplant shells and sprinkle over the feta.

Bake in the oven for 8–10 minutes or until the feta is melted and golden brown.

Tip

Want a vegan version? Use vegan feta instead. If you're not keen on soy mince and eat meat, use lean lamb or beef mince instead.

Low-carb nasi goreng

Gluten free • vegetarian • low carb • high protein • high fibre

SERVES: 2
PREP: 5 minutes
COOK: 10 minutes

Ingredients

2 tbsp coconut oil

3 garlic cloves, crushed

2 tbsp finely chopped ginger

½ onion, chopped

4 cups cauliflower rice

1 tbsp sesame oil

1 tbsp tamari sauce

4 eggs

½ green capsicum, chopped

1 baby red capsicum, chopped

2 tbsp freshly chopped coriander

sliced cucumber and cherry tomatoes, to serve

sesame seeds, to serve

Method

Preheat a wok on high heat.

Add 1 tablespoon of the coconut oil and when hot toss in the garlic, ginger and onion and fry for a few minutes. Add the riced cauliflower, sesame oil, tamari sauce and two of the eggs and mix vigorously until the eggs are cooked. Add the capsicum and fry for another 2–3 minutes then remove from heat.

In a separate pan heat the remaining tablespoon of coconut oil and fry the eggs until cooked to your liking.

Plate up the fried rice and top with fried egg, fresh coriander, cucumber, tomatoes and sesame seeds.

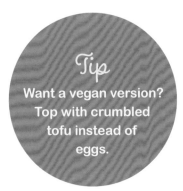

Tip
Want a vegan version? Top with crumbled tofu instead of eggs.

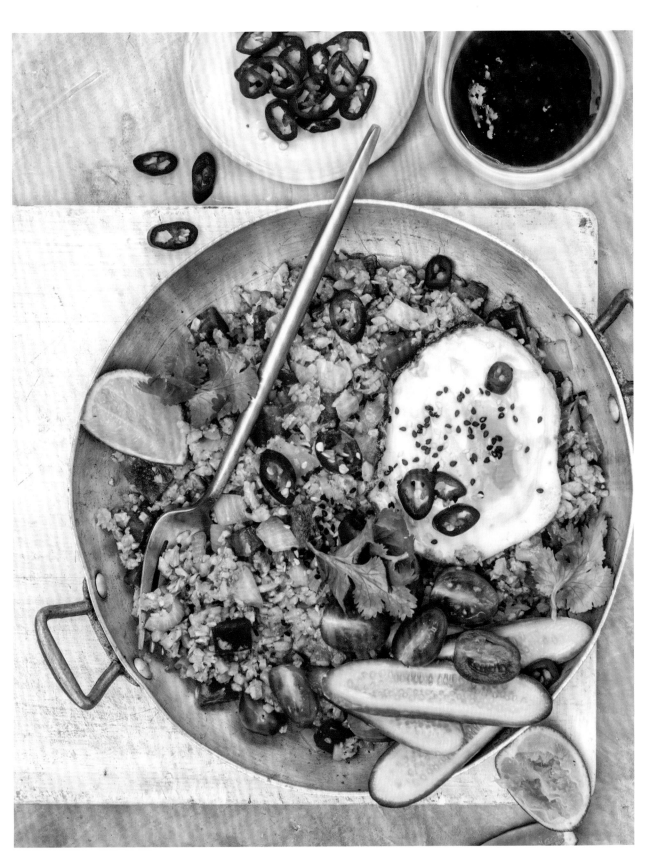

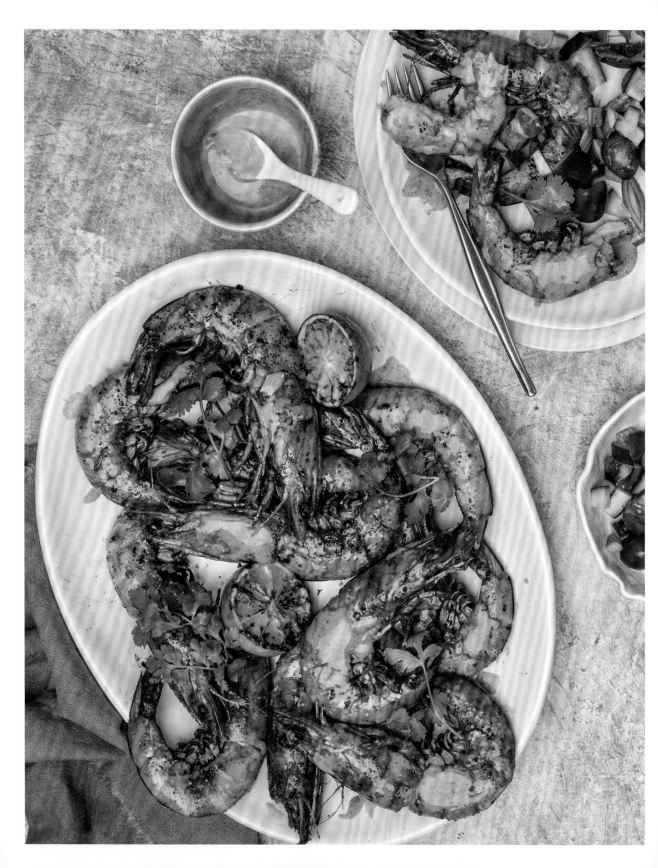

BBQ prawns

Gluten free • low carb • high protein
• keto-friendly

SERVES: 4
PREP: 5 minutes
COOK: 10 minutes

Ingredients

300 g fresh raw green
    prawns, unpeeled
1 tbsp olive oil
1 tsp minced garlic
1 tsp smoked paprika
½ tsp Italian seasoning
1 tsp onion powder
1 tsp garlic powder
salt and pepper, to taste
1 tbsp butter
2 tbsp coconut cream

Method

Preheat a BBQ grill or a chargrill pan over medium heat.

In a bowl mix the prawns with the olive oil, garlic, smoked paprika, Italian seasoning, onion powder, garlic powder and salt and pepper to season. Mix until prawns are well coated.

Grill the prawns for about 4 minutes each side until the skin is pink and the flesh is cooked through.

If cooking on a chargrill pan, add the butter and cream to the prawns to make a rich sauce. If cooking on a BBQ, heat a frying pan over the flame and add the butter, cream and prawns and stir until well combined.

Tip

This dish goes well with a Greek salad and some roasted sweet potatoes for extra fibre and nutrients.

Low-carb chow mein

Gluten free • low carb • high protein
• keto-friendly

SERVES: 4
PREP: 5 minutes
COOK: 5 minutes

Ingredients

2 tbsp vegetable oil

500 g chicken thigh cut into strips

250 g broccoli florets

4 garlic cloves, minced

2 baby red capsicums, sliced

400 g konjac noodles

1 cup beansprouts

½ cup roasted cashews

½ long green shallot (spring onion), chopped

2 tsp tamari sauce

2 tsp sesame oil

Method

Heat a wok over high heat and add the vegetable oil and chicken strips and fry until golden, about 3 minutes. Transfer to a plate and set aside.

Add the broccoli, garlic, capsicum and noodles and fry until tender. Return the chicken to the pan along with the beansprouts, cashews, spring onion, tamari sauce and sesame oil and cook for another 1–2 minutes.

Serve immediately.

Tip

Want a vegan version? Use firm tofu or tempeh instead of chicken. If you're looking for a pescatarian version, use salmon chunks instead.

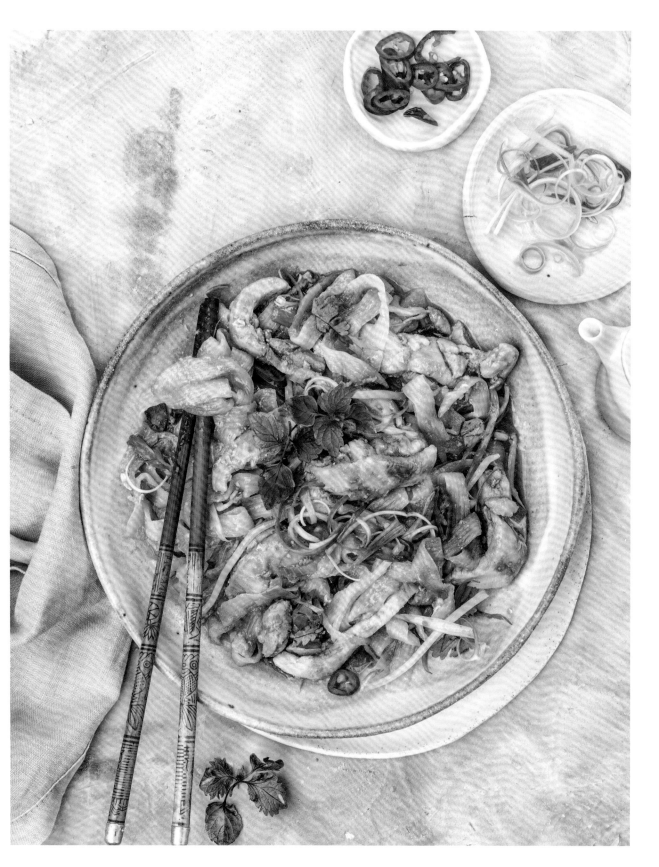

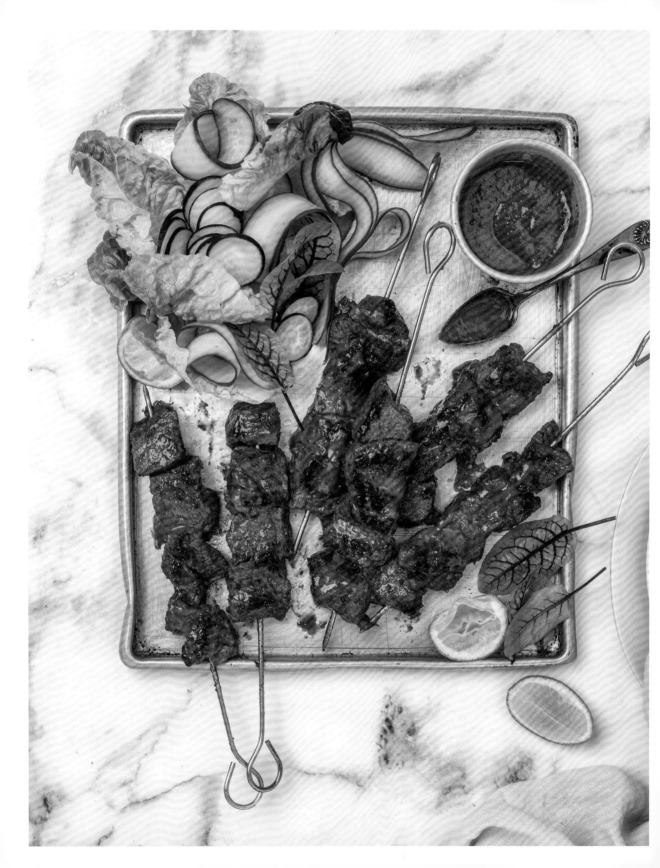

Easy satay salad

Gluten free • vegan • low carb • high protein • keto-friendly

SERVES: 4
PREP: 5 minutes
COOK: 5 minutes

Ingredients

- ½ cup unsweetened peanut butter
- ½ coconut milk
- ¼ cup water
- 2 tbsp tamari sauce
- 1 tsp vegan fish sauce
- 3 tsp freshly minced garlic
- 1 tsp freshly grated ginger
- 2 tsp fresh lemon juice
- 400 g tempeh, cut into 3-cm chunks
- 8 leaves oakleaf lettuce
- 2 Lebanese cucumbers peeled into ribbon
- 4 radishes, thinly sliced

Method

Whisk the peanut butter, coconut milk, water, tamari, fish sauce, garlic and ginger to make the satay sauce.

Preheat a BBQ grill or a chargrill pan over medium heat.

Thread the tempeh onto four small metal skewers. Brush the satay mixture over the kebabs and grill for about 5 minutes, turning to ensure they cook evenly.

Place remaining satay mixture in a saucepan and cook over a low heat for 2 minutes or so.

Drizzle skewers with remaining sauce and serve with the lettuce, cucumber and radish.

Tip

Want a meat version? Use lean fillet steak chunks instead of tempeh. Alternatively, this recipe works well with salmon chunks too, which will up your omega-3 intake.

DINNERS

Air-fryer wings

Gluten free • low carb • high protein

• keto-friendly

SERVES: 4
PREP: 5 minutes
COOK: 20 minutes

Ingredients

4 tbsp garlic powder

4 tbsp olive oil

salt and pepper, to taste

4 tbsp smoked paprika

1 cup grated parmesan cheese

16 chicken wings, skin-on

Method

In a medium bowl mix the garlic powder with the olive oil, salt and pepper, smoked paprika, and parmesan. Toss the wings in the mixture making sure each one is well coated.

Pop the wings in the air fryer at 180°C for about 20 minutes until the skin is golden and crispy, ensuring you flip them halfway through.

Transfer to a wire rack and let sit for 5 or so minutes before serving.

Tip

Serve these wings with a shaved fennel and rocket salad to up your daily veggie intake.

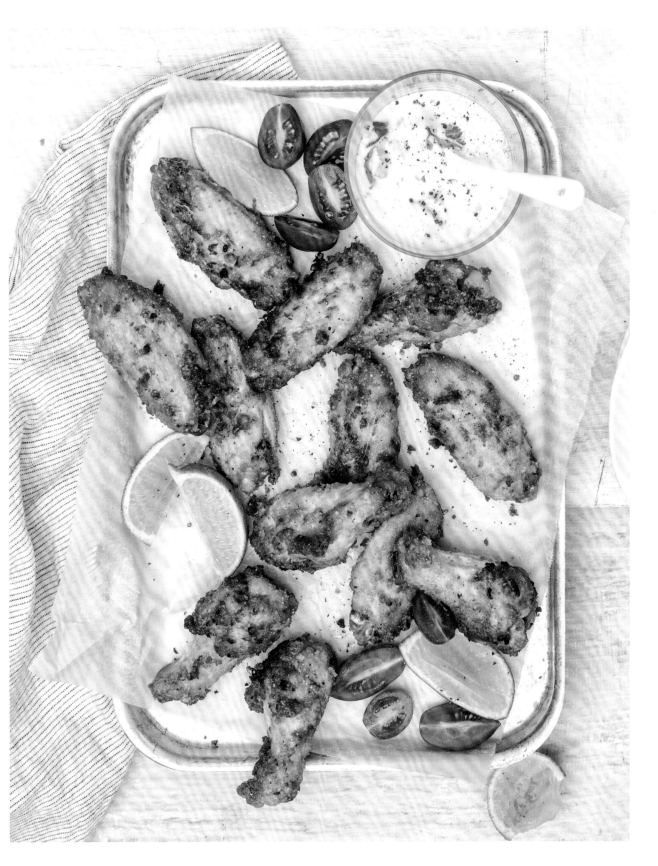

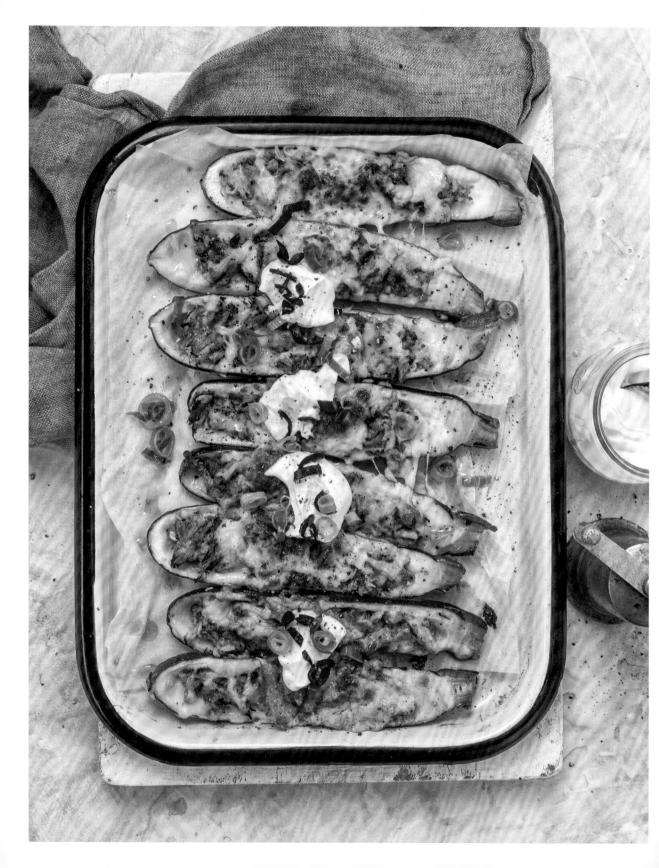

Zucchini boats

*Gluten free • vegan • low carb • high protein
• keto-friendly*

SERVES: 4
PREP: 5 minutes
COOK: 20 minutes

Ingredients

4 large zucchini, halved lengthwise

4 tsp olive oil

2 cups tempeh, shredded

1 tsp vegan sour cream

1 tsp tomato paste

1 tsp diced long green shallot (spring onion)

2 cups grated vegan cheddar cheese

sour cream, to serve

Method

Preheat the oven to 220°C. Line a baking tray with baking paper.

Hollow out the zucchini halves and brush with olive oil. Put the zucchini on the baking tray and bake in the oven for 10 minutes.

Meanwhile, mix the shredded tempeh, sour cream, tomato paste and spring onion in a bowl until well combined.

Remove the zucchini from the oven and stuff with the tempeh mixture. Top with grated cheese and bake for a further 10 minutes until the cheese is melted and golden brown.

Serve with a little sour cream.

Tip

Want a non-vegan version? Sub the tempeh for shredded chicken or tinned salmon to up your omega-3 intake.

DINNERS

Spinach pasta

Gluten free • vegetarian • low carb • high protein • keto-friendly

SERVES: 2
PREP: 10 minutes
COOK: 10 minutes

Ingredients

75 g lupin flour

30 g almond meal

½ tsp xanthan gum

pinch of ground nutmeg

1 tsp salt

1 egg

30 g water

25 g butter

1 bunch baby asparagus, halved lengthwise

1 garlic clove, minced

60 ml soy milk

100 g ricotta

2 tbsp lemon juice

salt and pepper, to taste

1 cup spinach

25 g grated parmesan cheese

Method

Put the lupin flour, almond meal, xanthan gum, nutmeg, egg and water in a food processor and pulse until a ball of dough forms.

Remove the dough from the food processor and roll out between two sheets of baking paper until less than 5-mm thick. Cut into thin tagliatelle, cook in a large pot of boiling water for 5 minutes and drain.

Melt the butter in a medium-sized pan over a medium heat. Add the asparagus and garlic and cook for around 3 minutes until tender. Add the milk, ricotta, lemon juice and salt and pepper to season.

Toss the spinach tagliatelle in the sauce, stir through the spinach, and top with parmesan before serving.

Tip
Want a vegan version? Use pulse pasta instead and sub the ricotta and parmesan for vegan substitutes.

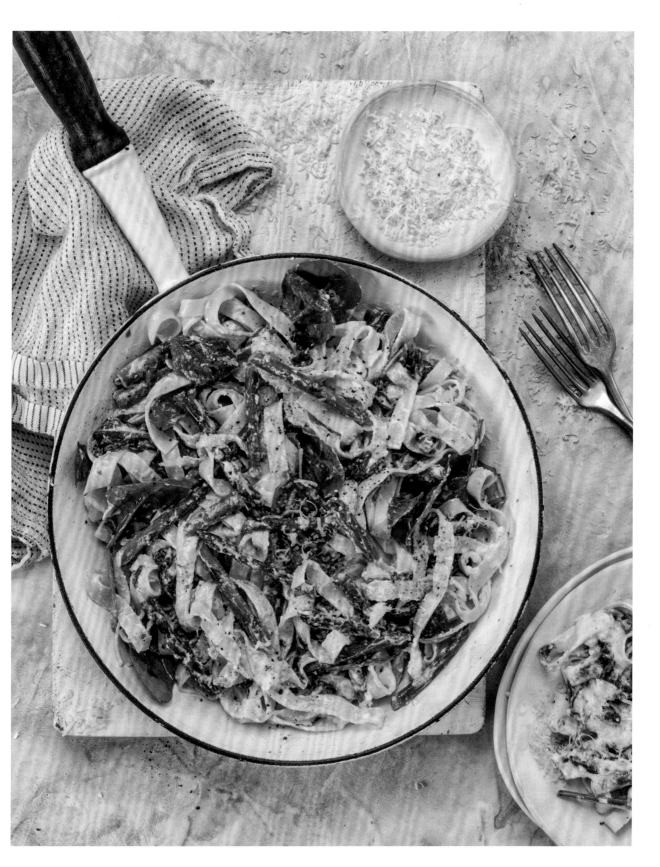

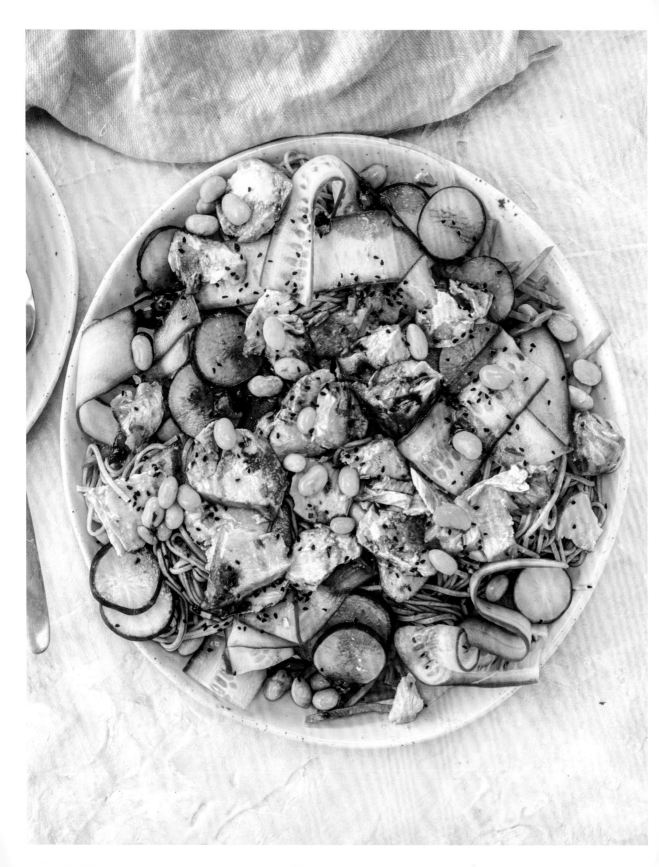

Salmon noodle bowl

Gluten free • high protein • high fibre

SERVES: 4
PREP: 10 minutes
COOK: 10 minutes

Ingredients

3 skinless salmon fillets

250 g soba noodles

¼ cup lime juice

2 tbsp vegetable oil

1 tbsp rice wine vinegar

2 tsp tamari sauce

1 tsp sesame oil

1 Lebanese cucumber
    cut into ribbons

100 g edamame, cooked

1 carrot, peeled and
    cut into matchsticks

2 long green shallots (spring
    onions), chopped

3 radishes, thinly sliced

toasted sesame seeds

Method

Bake the salmon fillets in the oven at 180°C for around 7 minutes until tender. Let rest for 5 minutes before flaking with a fork.

Cook noodles according to instructions on the packet, drain and toss in a little sesame oil.

Mix the lime juice, vegetable oil, vinegar, soy sauce and sesame oil in a bowl. Toss in the cucumber, edamame, carrot, spring onions and radish and mix well so everything is well coated.

Top with flaked salmon and sesame seeds.

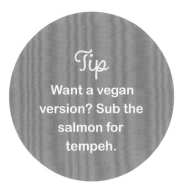

Tip
Want a vegan version? Sub the salmon for tempeh.

Asian turkey salad

Gluten free • high protein • high fibre

SERVES: 4
PREP: 10 minutes
COOK: 10 minutes

Ingredients

1 packet rice or egg noodles, cooked to instructions

1 skinless turkey breast, cooked and shredded

200 g snow peas, blanched

handful mint leaves, chopped

handful coriander leaves, chopped

3 long green shallots (spring onions), chopped

1 red chilli, chopped

1 cup coconut milk

¼ cup lime juice

1 tsp soy sauce

1 tsp sesame oil

1 tsp coconut sugar

Method

Toss the cooked noodles with the shredded turkey, snow peas, mint, coriander, spring onions and red chilli. Whisk together the coconut milk, lime juice, soy sauce, sesame oil and coconut sugar until well combined. Pour over the salad and mix well to coat.

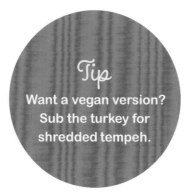

Tip

Want a vegan version? Sub the turkey for shredded tempeh.

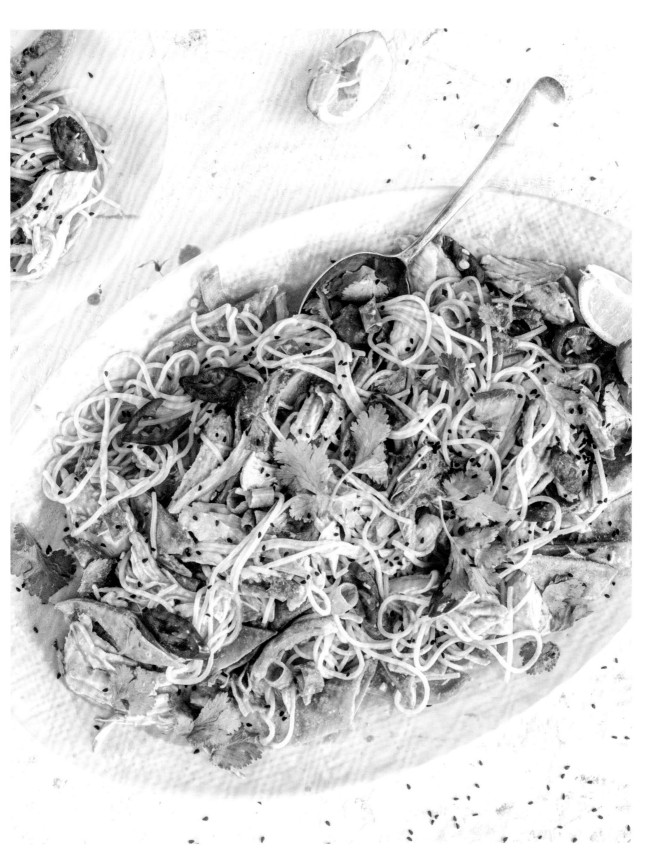

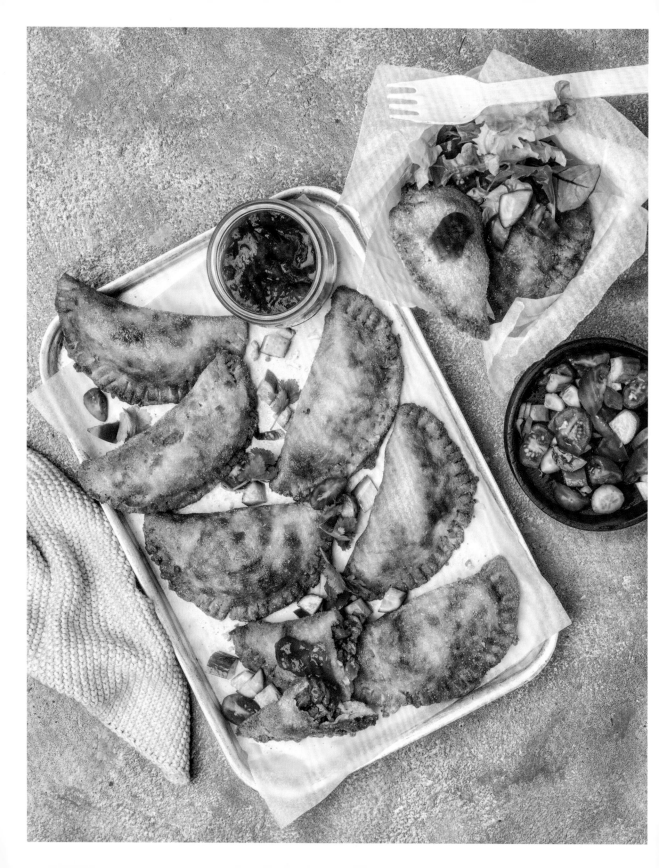

Low-carb empanadas

Gluten free • low carb • high protein • keto-friendly

SERVES: 2
PREP: 10 minutes
COOK: 10 minutes

Ingredients

1½ cups almond meal

2 eggs

3 cups mozzarella cheese

1 tbsp olive oil

¼ brown onion, diced

¼ red capsicum, diced

150 g turkey mince

½ tsp salt

½ tsp smoked paprika

¼ teaspoon ground cumin

½ tsp freshly ground pepper

extra olive oil for frying

Tip

Want a veggie version? Use plant-based soy mince instead of turkey. This also works well with minced salmon if you're looking for a pescatarian option.

Method

First make the dough by pulsing the almond meal with the eggs in a food processor until well combined.

In a microwave-proof bowl, melt the mozzarella cheese for a minute until smooth. Add the melted cheese to the mixture in the food processor and pulse again until a dough forms. Transfer to a bowl, cover with plastic wrap and refrigerate while you make the filling.

Heat a frying pan over medium heat and add the olive oil. Sauté the onion and red capsicum for 2–3 minutes or until softened. Add the mince and cook for 3–5 minutes until browned and breaking apart. Add the salt, smoked paprika, cumin and freshly ground pepper and cook for a minute or so until fragrant. Remove from the heat and allow to cool slightly.

Remove the dough from the fridge and roll out between two pieces of baking paper. Add a little cornflour if sticky. Roll until the dough is about 5-mm thick.

Use a round glass to cut out six circles. Place 1–2 tablespoons of filling into each circle, fold in half and crimp down the edges.

Heat another frying pan and shallow-fry the empanadas in olive oil for about 2–3 minutes until golden brown on each side.

DINNERS

Lentil moussaka

Gluten free • vegetarian • low carb • high protein

Ingredients

500 g eggplant, diced

2 tbsp olive oil

1 brown onion, chopped

2 garlic cloves, minced

1 tbsp ground cinnamon

1 tbsp smoked paprika

1 tsp dried oregano

1 tsp salt

400 g tin lentils

½ cup tomato passata

½ cup sour cream

6 tbsp cream cheese

2 cups grated mozzarella cheese

¼ tsp ground nutmeg

Method

Preheat the oven to 175°C.

Place a frying pan over a medium heat. Add the olive oil and eggplant and fry for about 5 minutes until soft. Add the onion, garlic, cinnamon, smoked paprika, oregano and salt and cook for another 5 minutes until the onion is translucent.

Add the lentils and cook for another 2–3 minutes. Stir in the tomato passata and simmer for 2 minutes or so.

In a separate saucepan over a medium heat mix the sour cream with the cream cheese, mozzarella cheese and nutmeg until a creamy sauce is formed.

Transfer the eggplant mixture to an ovenproof tray and top with the cheese sauce. Place in the oven and bake for 10 minutes or until cheese is golden and bubbling.

Tip

Want a vegan version?
Use vegan sour cream, cream cheese and mozzarella.
If you're after a meat version, use lean turkey mince.
Serve with a large Greek salad.

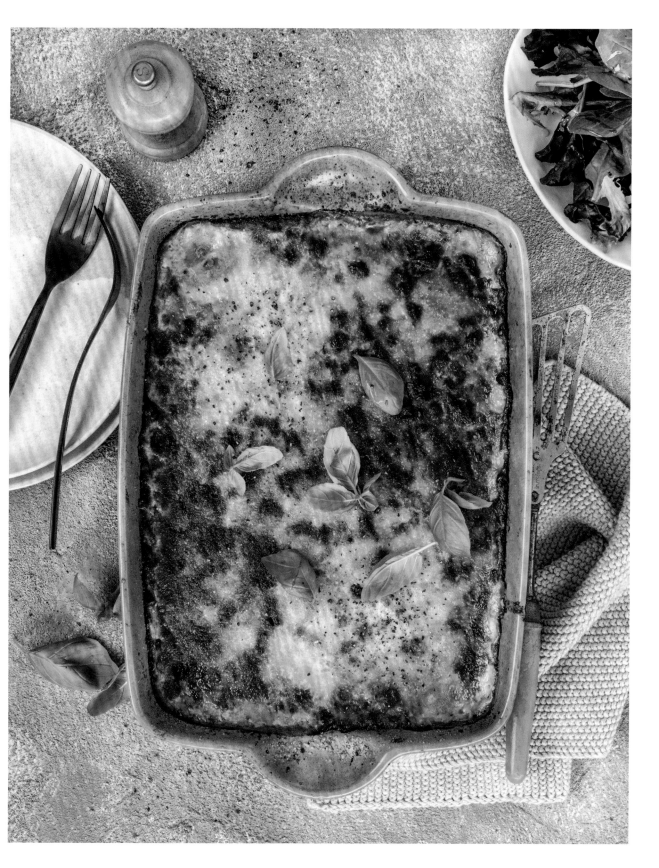

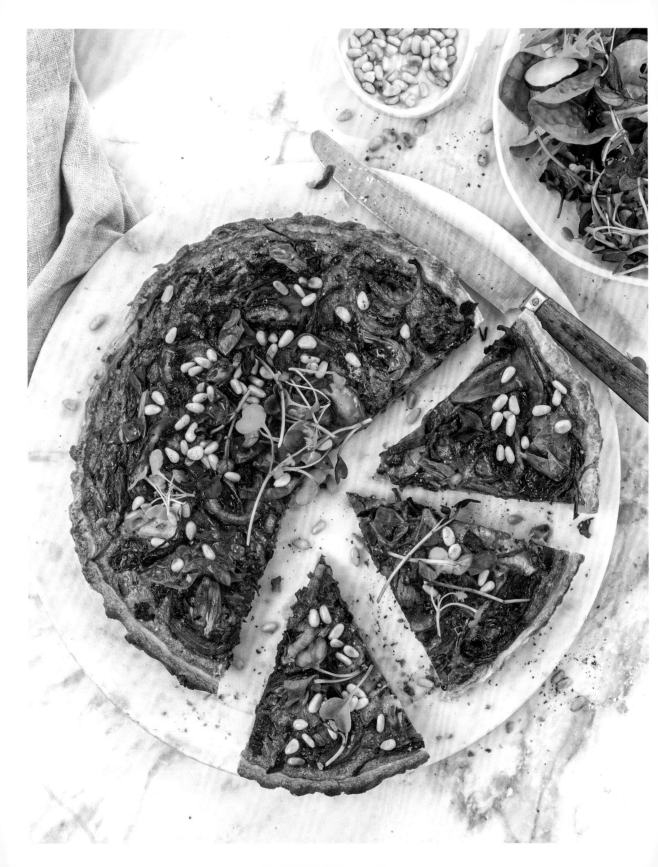

Vegan quiche

Gluten free • vegan • low carb • high protein

SERVES: 4
PREP: 10 minutes
COOK: 20 minutes

Ingredients

80 g of vegan butter, cubed

1 cup almond meal

pinch of salt

4 tablespoons cold water

1 red onion, chopped

punnet of mushrooms, chopped

1 clove garlic, crushed

350 g spinach, wilted and drained

350 g silken tofu

1 tsp chickpea flour

3 tbsp nutritional yeast

pinch of freshly ground nutmeg

½ teaspoon turmeric

salt and pepper, to taste

125 g vegan feta

toasted pine nuts, to serve

Method

Preheat the oven to 200°C.

Make the pastry by mixing the butter with the almond flour, salt, and water to form a dough. Roll out the pastry and gently press it into a quiche tin. Bake blind for 10 minutes then remove from oven.

Meanwhile, sauté the onion with the mushrooms and garlic until soft. Add the wilted spinach and set aside.

Make your egg replacement by blending the silken tofu, chickpea flour, nutritional yeast, ground nutmeg, turmeric, and salt and pepper.

Add the veggies and vegan feta to the pre-cooked pastry case and top with your tofu mixture.

Bake for 25–30 minutes until nicely set. Top with toasted pine nuts before serving.

Tip

Want a pescatarian version? Add in some smoked salmon for extra omega-3 intake.

DINNERS

Salmon bake

Low carb • high protein • high fibre

SERVES: 4
PREP: 10 minutes
COOK: 20 minutes

Ingredients

50 g butter

1 small brown onion, diced

2 sticks celery, diced

250 g mushrooms, diced

3 cloves garlic, minced

50 g cream cheese

¼ cup sour cream

¼ cup soy milk

½ cup grated mozzarella cheese

200 g tin salmon

salt and pepper, to taste

1 stale sourdough roll

⅓ cup grated cheddar cheese

fresh parsley, to serve

Method

Preheat the oven to 180°C. Grease a casserole dish with a little butter.

Place a medium-sized saucepan over a medium heat and add the remaining butter, onion and celery and sauté for about 5 minutes until translucent. Add the mushrooms and garlic and cook for a further 5 minutes.

Add the sour cream, cream cheese and milk and bring to a simmer. Stir through the mozzarella cheese and remove the pan from the heat.

Add the salmon to the pan and stir through to combine. Season with salt and pepper to taste and then spoon into the casserole dish. Top with the torn sourdough roll and sprinkle the cheddar cheese on top.

Bake in the oven for 15–20 minutes until the cheese is melted and bubbling and the bread is golden brown.

Tip
This recipe also works well with tinned tuna. Serve with a watercress salad.

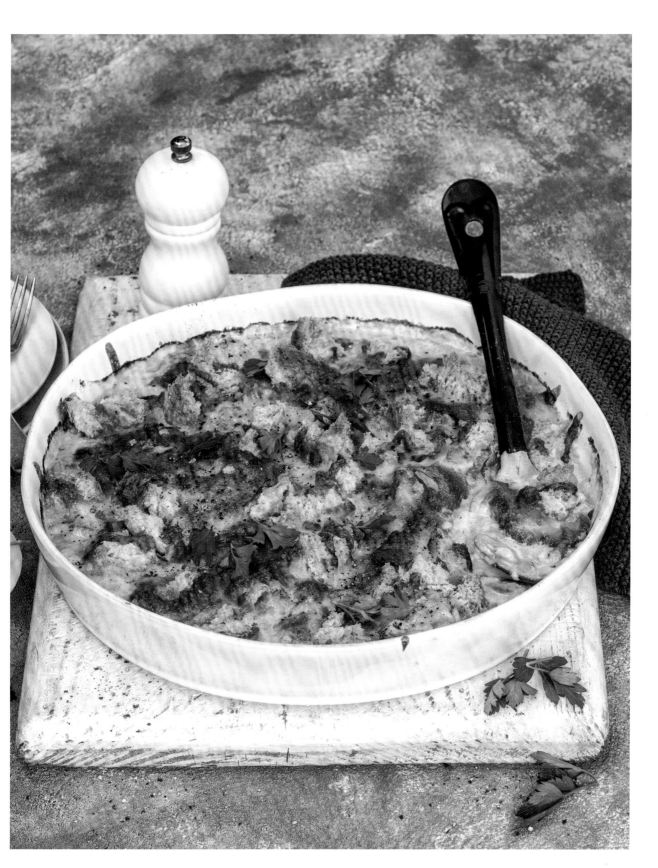

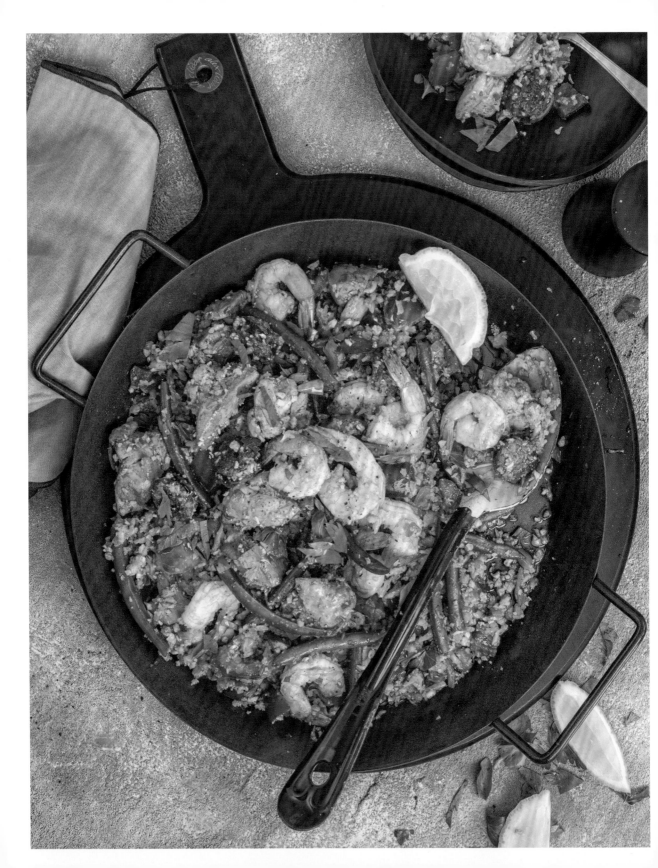

Low-carb paella

Gluten free • low carb • high protein
• keto-friendly

SERVES: 4
PREP: 10 minutes
COOK: 10 minutes

Ingredients

5 cups cauliflower rice

2 tbsp olive oil

2 chicken skinless thighs, deboned and diced

70 g chorizo, sliced

1 brown onion, diced

2 cloves garlic, crushed

1 red capsicum, diced

150 g fresh prawns

½ cup chicken stock

1 ripe tomato, diced

½ cup green beans

1 tbsp smoked paprika

salt and pepper, to taste

½ tsp saffron threads or ground saffron

½ lemon

fresh parsley, chopped, to serve

Method

First grate your cauliflower and set aside.

Heat the olive oil in a medium-sized frying pan over a medium heat and sear the chicken and chorizo for around 5 minutes each side. Remove from the pan and set aside.

In the same pan sauté the onion, garlic and capsicum for about 2–3 minutes until translucent then add the prawns.

Return the chicken and chorizo to the pan and add the cauliflower rice, stock, tomato, green beans, smoked paprika, salt and pepper and saffron and cook for a further 5 minutes.

Serve topped with a squeeze of lemon juice and parsley.

Tip

Want a vegan version? Sub the chicken and chorizo for tempeh and the prawns for artichoke hearts and add some frozen peas for additional protein.

Cod tray bake

Gluten free • low carb • high protein • keto-friendly

SERVES: 2
PREP: 10 minutes
COOK: 25 minutes

Ingredients

1 head cauliflower cut into 2-cm florets

3 tbsp olive oil

salt and pepper, to taste

½ tsp smoked paprika

2 cod fillets, or other firm white fish

1 tbsp harissa paste

150 g cherry tomatoes, quartered

juice of ½ a lime

2 tsp freshly chopped coriander

Method

Preheat the oven to 220°C and line a baking tray with baking paper.

Put the cauliflower florets on the tray and massage in 1 tablespoon of olive oil, salt, pepper and paprika and roast for about 15 minutes.

Season the cod with harissa and rub in the rest of the olive oil.

Remove cauliflower from the oven and place the cod in the centre of the tray and cook for a further 10 minutes.

Meanwhile, mix the cherry tomatoes, lime juice and coriander in a bowl and set aside.

Remove the fish from the oven and serve with the cauliflower and tomatoes.

Tip

Want a vegan version? Sub the cod for firm tofu steaks. Make sure the tofu is nice and dry and score it before rubbing in the harissa.

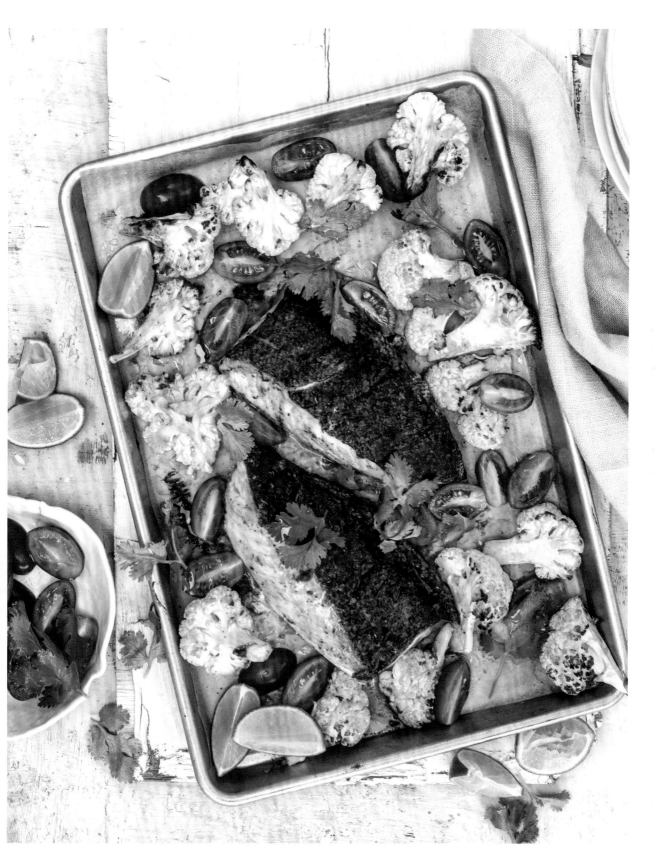

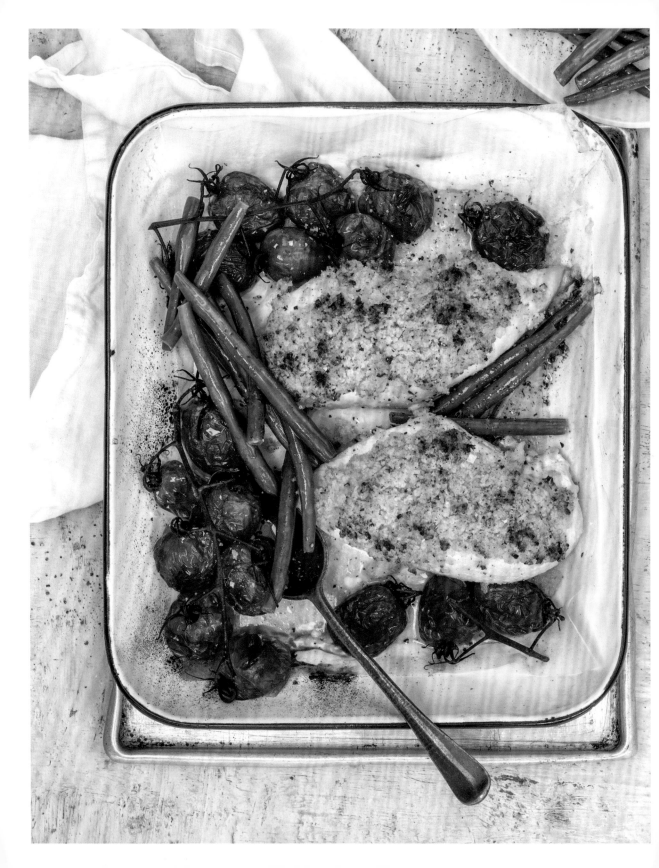

Chicken Kiev

High fibre • low carb • high protein

Ingredients

4 chicken breasts

80 g butter, melted

3 cloves garlic, minced

2 tsp freshly chopped
    parsley

1 small lemon, zested
    and cut into quarters

salt and pepper, to taste

1 stale sourdough bun,
    processed into
    breadcrumbs

250 g truss cherry tomatoes

250 g green beans, trimmed

drizzle of olive oil

Method

Preheat the oven to 220°C and line a baking tray
with baking paper. Place the chicken on the tray.

Mix the butter, garlic, parsley, lemon zest and salt
and pepper in a bowl until well combined.

Pour half the mixture over the chicken. Add the
breadcrumbs to the other half of the mixture then press
the breadcrumbs on the top of the chicken. Place the
tomatoes and green beans around the chicken and
drizzle with olive oil.

Bake for 20 minutes and serve with leafy greens
and lemon wedges.

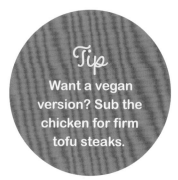

Tip
Want a vegan
version? Sub the
chicken for firm
tofu steaks.

Mushroom risotto

Gluten free • vegetarian • low carb • high protein

SERVES: 2
PREP: 5 minutes
COOK: 10 minutes

Ingredients

1 tbsp butter

1 French shallot, diced

2 garlic cloves, minced

150g button mushrooms, quartered

½ a large cauliflower, riced

½ cup veggie stock

½ cup sour cream

¼ cup grated parmesan cheese

salt and pepper, to taste

freshly chopped parsley and toasted pumpkin seeds, to serve

Method

Melt the butter in a medium frying pan over a medium heat. Add the shallot and garlic and sauté for 2–3 minutes until softened. Add the mushrooms and fry for 5 minutes until soft and tender. Add the riced cauliflower and cook for another 2 minutes. Pour in the stock and let simmer for another 5 minutes until the liquid is absorbed. Stir in the sour cream and cook for another 2 minutes.

Remove from the heat and stir in the parmesan cheese and salt and pepper to taste. Top with a sprinkle of toasted pumpkin seeds and some freshly chopped parsley before serving.

Tip

Want a vegan version? Sub the sour cream and parmesan for vegan alternatives. Eat meat? Add some diced chicken for an extra protein boost.

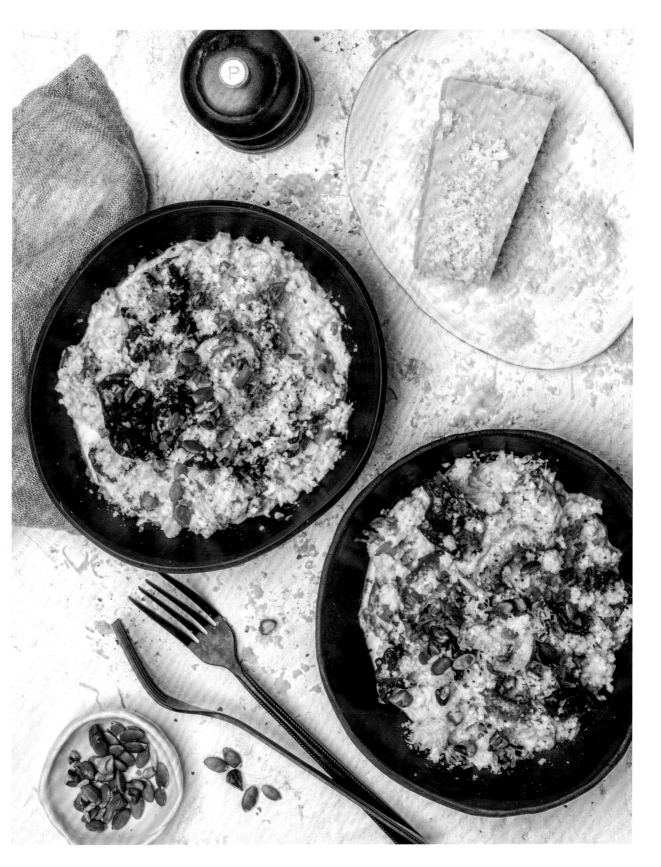

Zucchini
choc-chip muffins
Healthy Cherry Ripe
Fluffy low-carb rolls
Low-carb orange cake
Lemon and blueberry cake
Mango cheesecake
Matcha ice cream
Apple popsicles
Vegan pavs
Green smoothie
Turmeric latte cookies
Orange cardamom sorbet
Raspberry slice
Lemon seed muffins
Passionfruit cheesecake
Protein mocha pops
Gluten-free summer puddings
Low-carb black forest cake
Parmesan prawn tacos
Kefir sorbet

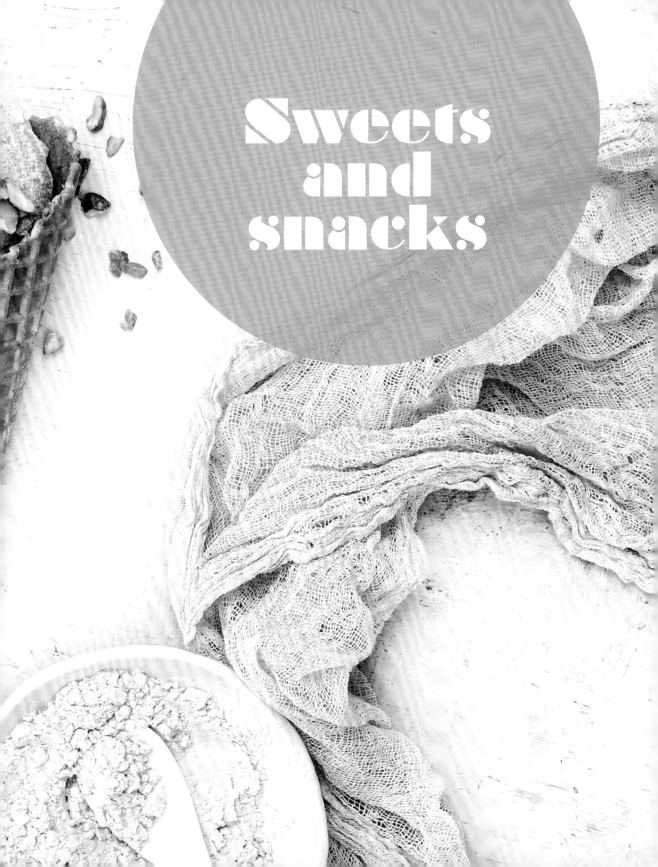

Sweets and snacks

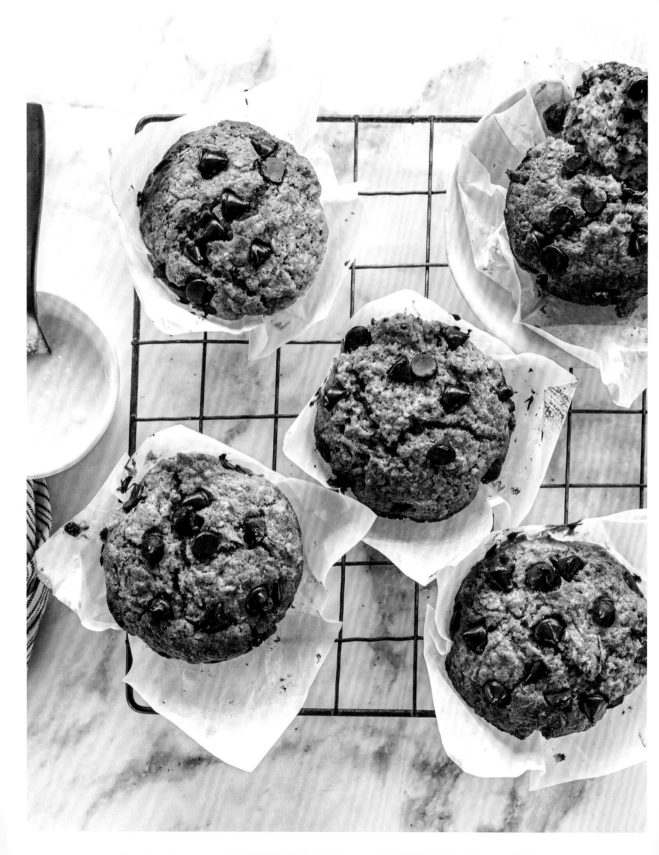

Zucchini choc-chip muffins

Gluten free • vegetarian • low carb • high protein

MAKES: 12
PREP: 5 minutes
COOK: 15 minutes

Ingredients

1½ cups grated zucchini

1¼ cups almond meal

1 cup gluten-free oats

1 tsp cinnamon

¼ tsp allspice

¼ tsp nutmeg

1 tbsp baking powder

½ tsp salt

½ cup maple syrup

1 tsp vanilla

1 cup kefir

¼ cup coconut oil, melted

2 eggs

⅓ cup dark sugar-free
    mini chocolate chips

Method

Preheat the oven to 180°C. Line a muffin tin with muffin cases.

Grate the zucchini over a tea towel and squeeze to remove excess water.

Combine the dry ingredients in a bowl. Combine the wet ingredients in a large mixing bowl. Whisk until well combined. Gradually, add the dry ingredients to the wet ingredients. Fold in the zucchini and chocolate chips.

Fill the muffin cases about three-quarters full. Bake for 10–15 minutes. Check at 10 minutes to see if a skewer comes out clean.

Tip

Want a vegan version? Sub the eggs for one banana or 2 tablespoons of apple sauce, and the kefir for soy yoghurt.

Healthy Cherry Ripe

Gluten free • vegan • low carb • high protein

MAKES: 12
PREP: 75 minutes

Ingredients

2 cups desiccated coconut

3 tbsp coconut oil

3 tbsp coconut sugar

1 teaspoon vanilla extract

1 cup frozen pitted cherries

⅓ cup frozen raspberries

200 g 85% dark chocolate

Method

Line a 20 cm square tin with baking paper.

Blend the coconut, oil, coconut sugar and vanilla extract in a food processor until well combined. Add the cherries and raspberries to the mixture and pulse until well combined.

Press mixture into the prepared tin and place in the freezer for one hour. Remove from the freezer and cut into 12 equal bars.

Melt chocolate in the microwave and stir vigorously until smooth. Dip bars one by one in the melted chocolate and sit them on a wire rack to set.

Store bars in the fridge and once set place in an airtight container.

Tip

Want a keto-friendly version? Sub the coconut sugar for monkfruit extract or stevia.

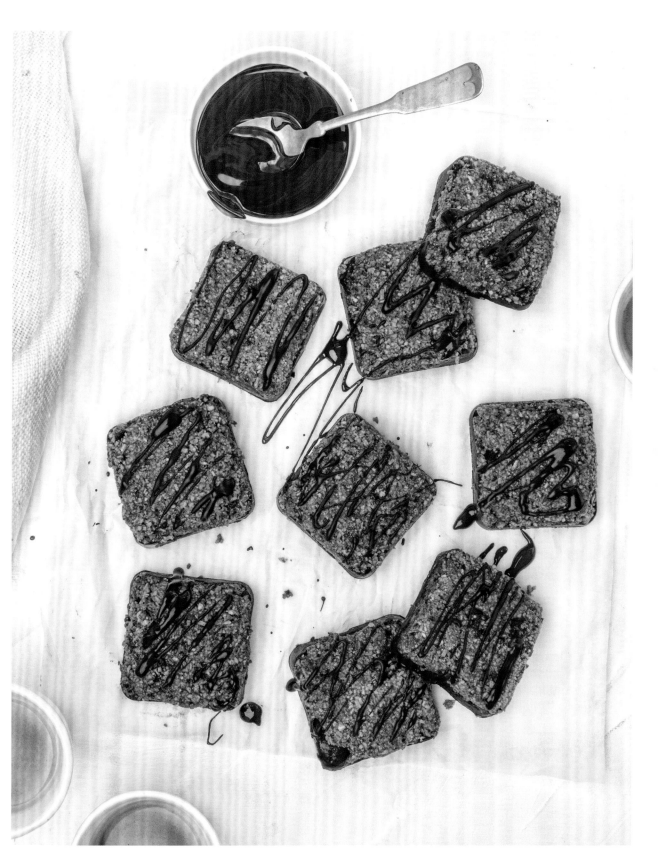

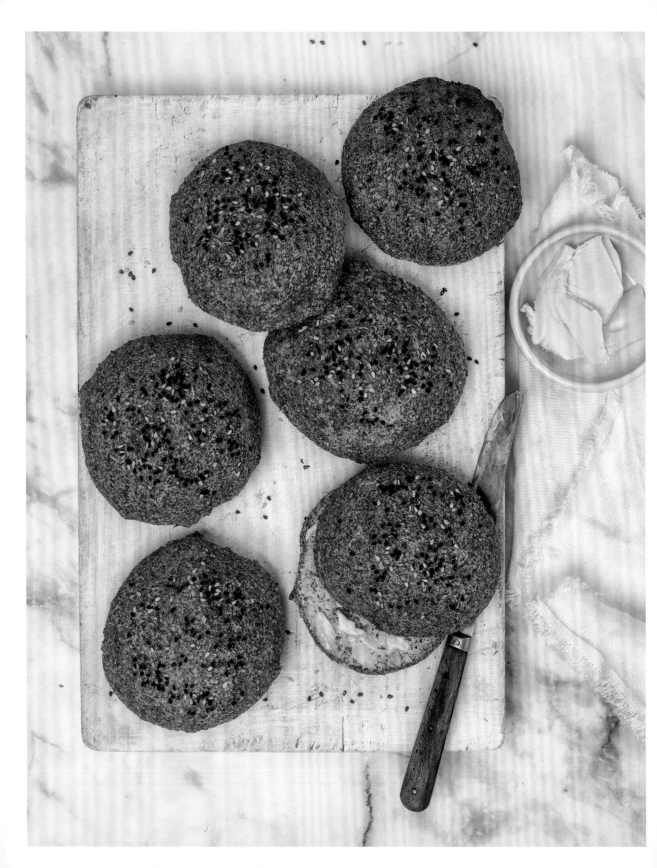

Fluffy low-carb rolls

Gluten free • vegetarian • low carb • high protein

MAKES: 4
PREP: 5 minutes
COOK: 30 minutes

Ingredients

1 cup almond meal

2 tbsp psyllium husk

1 tsp bicarb (baking) soda

1 tbsp apple cider vinegar

½ cup boiling water

2 egg whites

sesame seeds

Method

Preheat the oven to 180°C. Line a baking tray with baking paper.

Combine the almond flour with the psyllium husk and bicarb soda in a medium bowl. Add the apple cider vinegar, boiling water and egg whites and mix to form a gooey dough.

Split dough into two pieces, roll into bread rolls and top with sesame seeds.

Place on the baking tray and bake for 30 minutes until golden brown, the bottom is crisp and the bread roll sounds hollow when tapped.

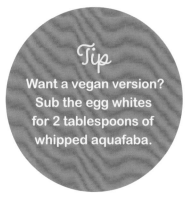

Tip

Want a vegan version? Sub the egg whites for 2 tablespoons of whipped aquafaba.

Low-carb orange cake

Gluten free • vegetarian • low carb • high protein

SERVES: *8*
PREP: *5 minutes*
COOK: *30 minutes*

Ingredients

2 whole boiled oranges,
   pips removed

2 cups almond meal

1 cup maple syrup

1 tsp vanilla extract

6 eggs, separated

1 tub coconut yoghurt

1 tsp vanilla extract

3 tbsp maple syrup

chopped almonds

Method

Preheat oven to 180°C. Grease and line a 20 cm springform cake tin.

Put the boiled and cooled whole oranges, almond meal, maple syrup, vanilla extract and egg yolks in the blender and blend until smooth.

Whisk egg whites until stiff and fold into the batter. Bake for about an hour or until a skewer comes out clean.

Once the cake is cool, whisk the yoghurt with the vanilla extract and maple syrup until creamy. Frost cake and top with almonds.

Tip

Want a vegan version? Sub the eggs for 6 teaspoons whipped aquafaba.

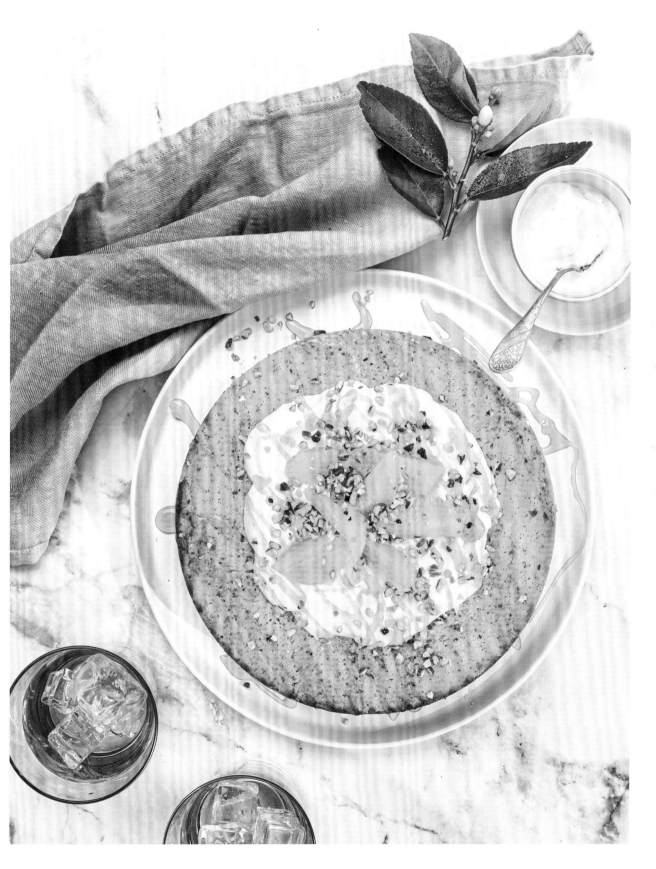

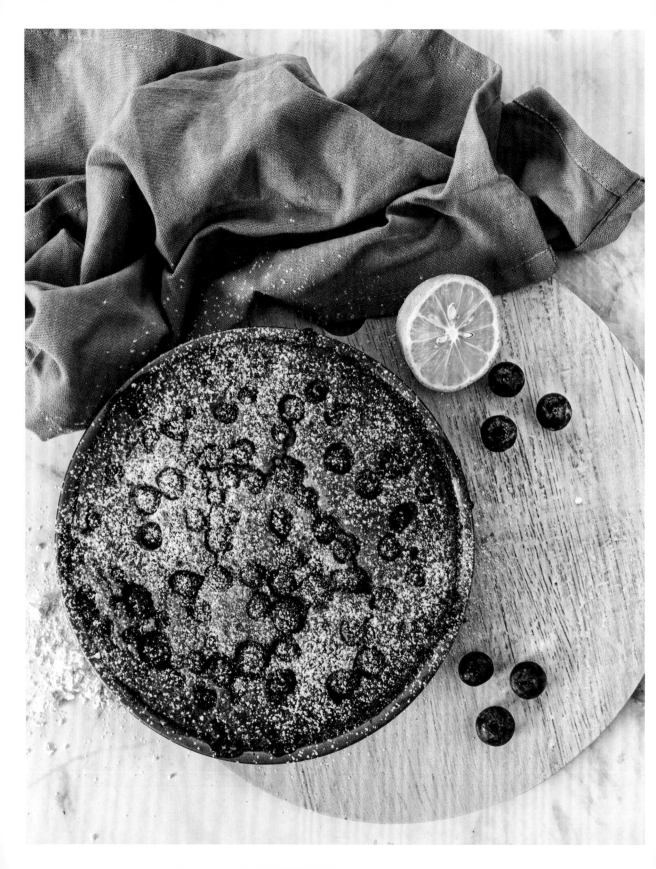

Lemon and blueberry cake

Gluten free • vegetarian • low carb • high protein • high fibre

SERVES: 8
PREP: 5 minutes
COOK: 30 minutes

Ingredients

3 large eggs

1 cup coconut sugar

1 cup coconut yoghurt

½ cup coconut oil, melted

1 tsp vanilla extract

¼ tsp salt

2 cups almond meal

1 cup oat flour

1 scoop vegan protein powder

2 tsp baking powder

zest and juice of 1 medium lemon

punnet of blueberries

Method

Preheat oven to 180°C. Grease a 20 cm cake tin.

Whisk eggs and coconut sugar together. Add the coconut yoghurt, oil, vanilla extract and salt. Fold in the almond meal, oat flour, protein powder, baking powder and whisk again until combined. Add the lemon zest and juice, whisk again until smooth then pour into the cake tin and top with the blueberries.

Bake for 30 minutes or until cooked through and springy to touch.

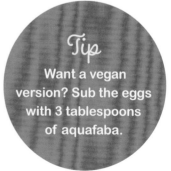

Tip
Want a vegan version? Sub the eggs with 3 tablespoons of aquafaba.

Mango cheesecake

Gluten free • vegetarian • low carb • high protein • keto-friendly

SERVES: 8
PREP: 5 minutes
COOK: 30 minutes

Ingredients

250 g almond flour

100 g melted unsalted butter

100 g desiccated coconut

flesh of 3 mangoes, blended

2 tbsp monkfruit extract

500 g cream cheese

300 g Greek yoghurt

3 eggs, whisked

2 tsp vanilla extract

1 tbsp freshly grated
    turmeric

sliced fresh mango,
    to garnish

toasted coconut pieces,
    to garnish

Method

Preheat oven to 180°C.

Mix the almond flour with the melted butter and desiccated coconut. Press the mixture into a 30 cm springform cake tin and bake for 10 minutes until golden. Remove from the oven and let cool.

Reduce the oven temperature to 150°C.

Combine the mango, monkfruit extract, cream cheese, yoghurt, eggs, vanilla extract and grated turmeric and mix until smooth. Pour into the cake tin and bake the cheesecake for about an hour until set. Remove from the oven and leave to cool.

Once the cheesecake has cooled top with fresh mango and toasted coconut pieces.

Tip

Want a vegan version? Sub the butter, cream cheese and yoghurt for vegan alternatives and the eggs for aquafaba.

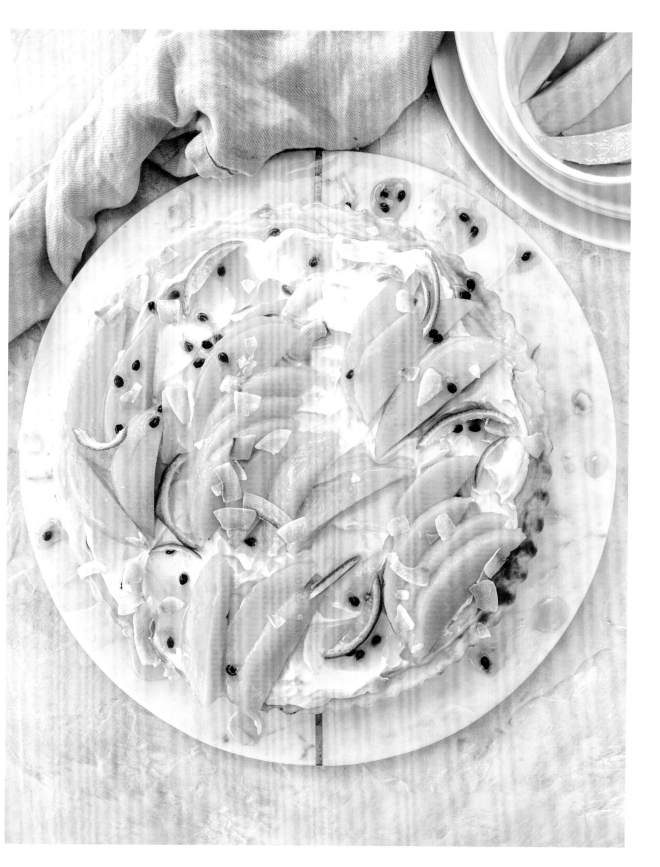

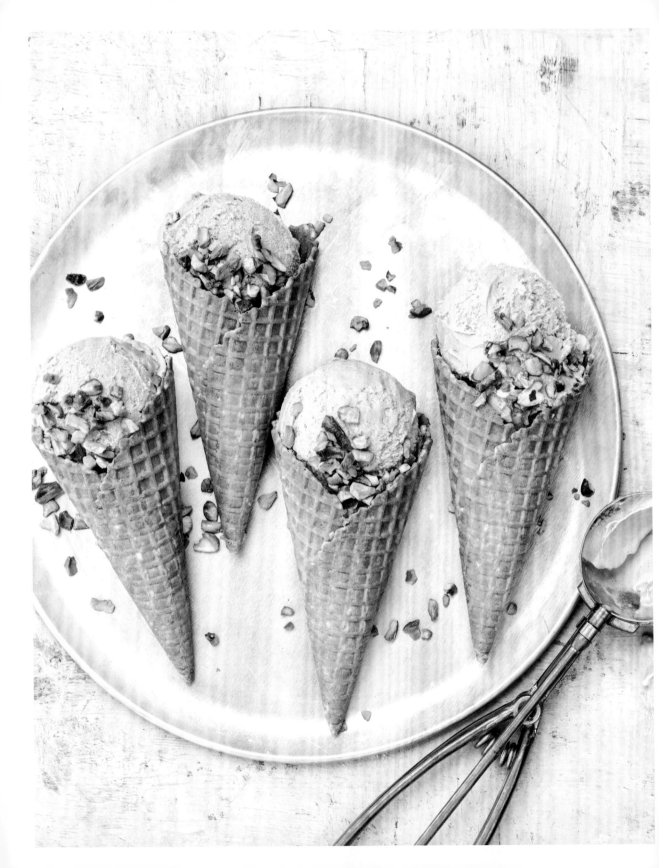

Matcha ice cream

Gluten free • vegan • low carb • high protein

SERVES: 6
PREP: 6–8 hours

Ingredients

1 cup soy milk

3 scoops vegan matcha tea protein powder

1 cup canned coconut milk

½ an avocado

Method

Blend the milk, protein powder, coconut milk and avocado in a blender until smooth. Transfer mix to an ice-cream maker and churn according to manufacturer's instructions. Freeze for at least 3 hours before serving.

Serve in a waffle cone with a sprinkle of pistachio nuts.

Tip

If you can't find matcha tea protein powder, simply mix 1 teaspoon of matcha tea with vegan vanilla protein powder.

Apple popsicles

Gluten free • vegan • low carb • keto-friendly

SERVES: 6
PREP: 6-8 hours

Ingredients

4 cups juiced green apples
½ cup lime juice
½ cup mint leaves
½ cup coconut cream

Method

Put the green apple juice, lime juice and mint leaves in a blender and blitz until smooth. Pour into popsicle moulds and top with coconut cream then freeze overnight.

Serve with toasted coconut for extra crunch.

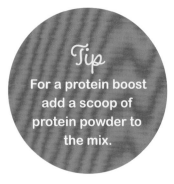

Tip
For a protein boost add a scoop of protein powder to the mix.

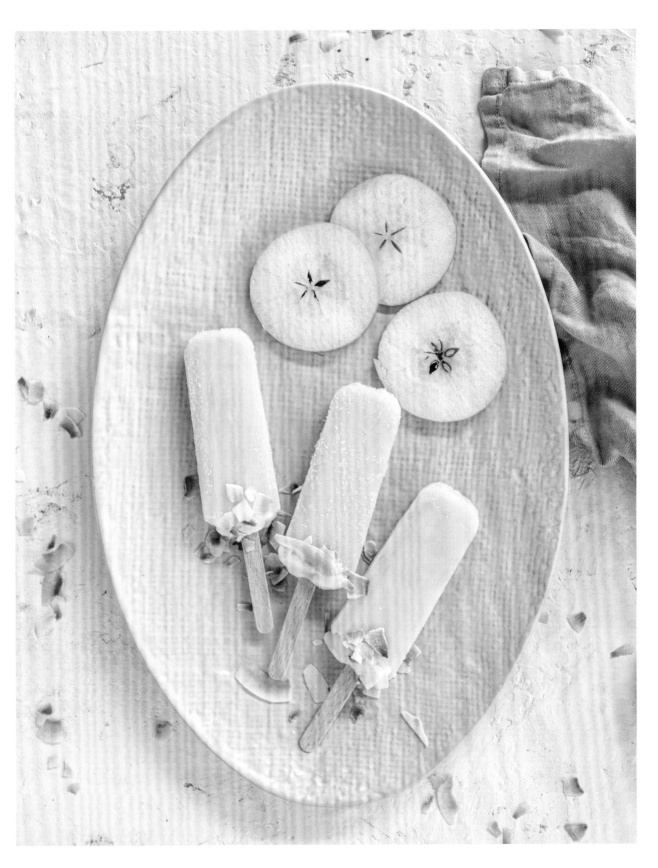

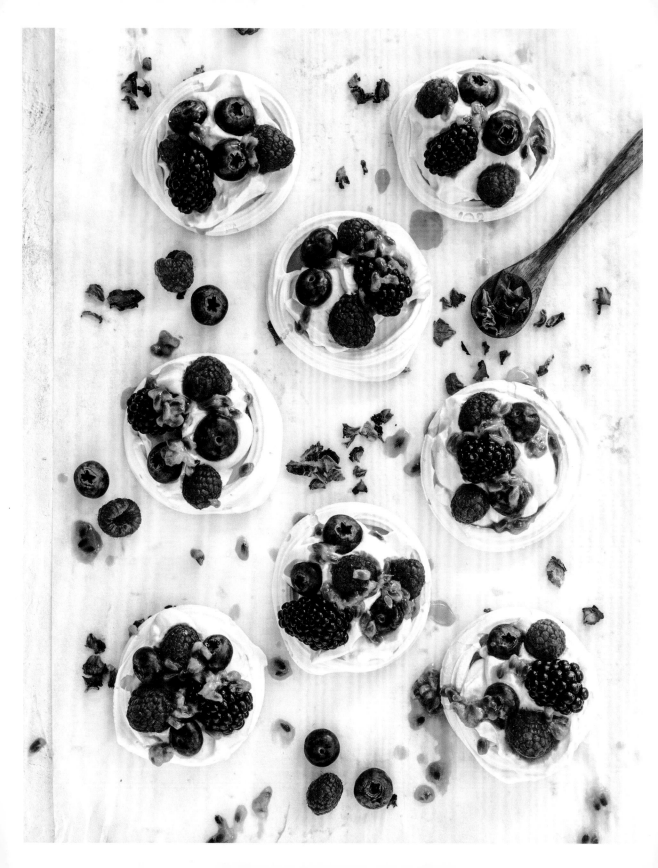

Vegan pavs

Gluten free • vegan • low carb • keto-friendly

SERVES: 6
PREP: 10 minutes
COOK: 60 minutes

Ingredients

400 ml can of chickpea water (aquafaba), chilled

½ cup monkfruit extract

1 tbsp cornflour

400 ml can coconut cream, chilled overnight

½ cup monkfruit powdered sweetener

1 tsp vanilla extract

1 punnet blueberries

1 punnet raspberries

1 punnet strawberries, hulled and quartered

passionfruit pulp, to drizzle

Tip
Want a non-vegan version? Just sub the aquafaba for six egg whites.

Method

Preheat the oven to 150°C. Line a large baking tray with baking paper.

Take the drained liquid from the chilled chickpeas (aquafaba) and place in a stand mixer and whip until soft peaks form. Add the monkfruit extract, one tablespoon at a time until dissolved. Add the cornflour and whisk until combined.

Dollop 12 rounds of the meringue mixture onto the baking tray and bake in the oven for around an hour or until the pavlovas are crisp and firm. Turn off the oven and let the meringues sit for a few hours.

Once cooled, remove the coconut cream from the fridge and remove the liquid before putting the cream in the bowl of a stand mixer. Whisk on high until stiff peaks form, then reduce to low speed, slowly adding the monkfruit powdered sweetener and vanilla extract.

Top the pavlovas with the coconut cream, berries and passionfruit pulp.

Green smoothie

Gluten free • vegetarian • gut-friendly • low carb • high fibre

SERVES: 2
PREP: 10 minutes

Ingredients

½ cup chopped mango

1 banana, chopped

1 thumb of ginger

1 lime, juiced

2 cups spinach

½ cup walnuts

1 cup kefir

1 cup coconut water

Method

Place all the ingredients in a blender with a little ice and blitz until smooth.

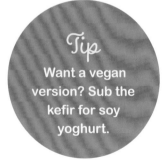

Tip
Want a vegan version? Sub the kefir for soy yoghurt.

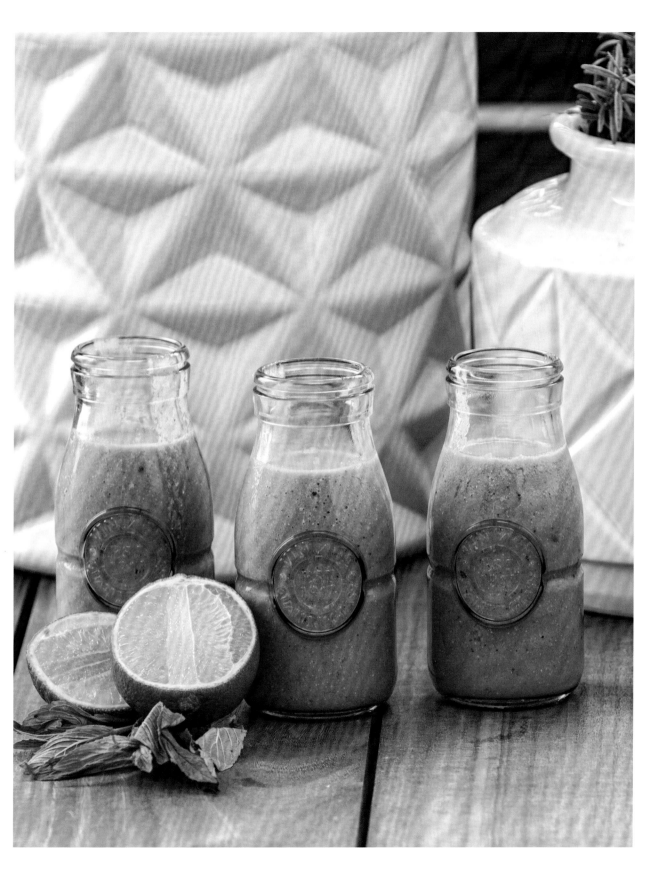

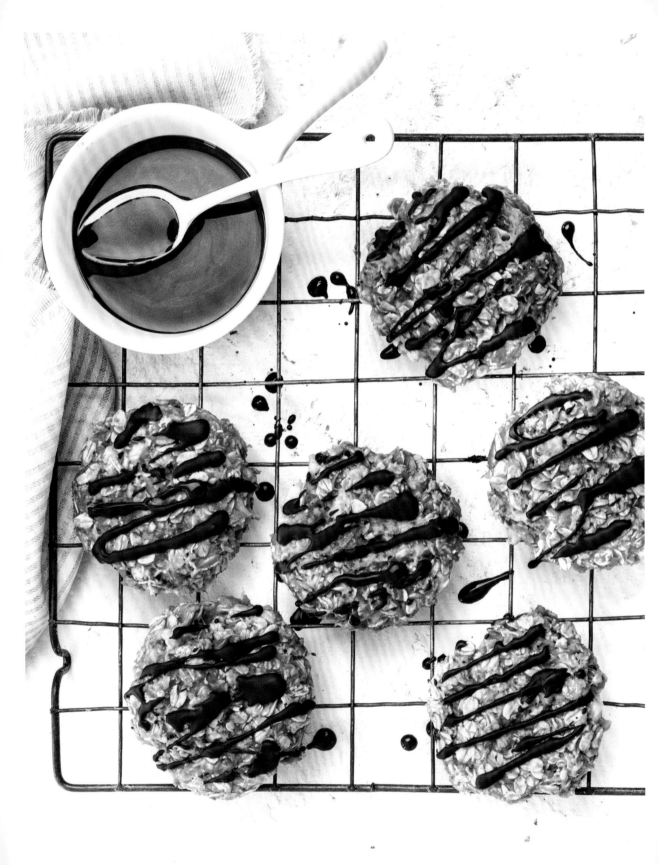

Turmeric latte cookies

Gluten free • vegetarian • gut-friendly • low carb • high fibre

PREP: 5 minutes
COOK: 15 minutes

Ingredients

2 cups gluten-free oats
1 scoop protein powder
1 tsp turmeric powder
½ cup cashew butter
½ cup soy milk
1 mashed banana
pinch of pink Himalayan salt
melted dark chocolate

Method

Preheat oven to 180°C. Line a baking tray with baking paper.

Combine the oats, protein powder and turmeric in a bowl and stir until well combined. Add the cashew butter, soy milk, mashed banana and salt and combine to make a dough. Shape into about 15 cookies and place on a baking tray with parchment paper. Bake for around 15 minutes, until golden.

Once cool drizzle with a little melted dark chocolate.

Tip
Want a keto version? Sub the oats for almond meal and the banana for an egg.

Orange cardamom sorbet

Gluten free • vegan • low carb

SERVES: 6
PREP: 6–8 hours

Ingredients

3 cups water

1 cup coconut sugar

½ cup manuka honey

2 tbsp fresh orange zest

1 tbsp grated ginger

2 cardamom pods

2 whole cloves

1 bay leaf

2 cups freshly squeezed orange juice

3 tbsp freshly squeezed lemon juice

Method

Combine the water, coconut sugar, honey, orange zest, grated ginger, cardamom, cloves and bay leaf in a heavy-based saucepan. Bring to the boil over medium–high heat, stirring until the sugar dissolves. Boil until the syrup is thick and mixture is reduced to about 2 cups (around 10–12 minutes), then discard the bay leaf and let the syrup cool.

Strain syrup into a bowl. Add the orange juice and lemon juice then transfer to an ice-cream maker and process in accordance with the manufacturer's instructions.

Transfer the sorbet to a container, cover and freeze until firm, for at least 6 hours before serving.

Tip

For a protein boost add two scoops of vegan vanilla protein powder to the mix.

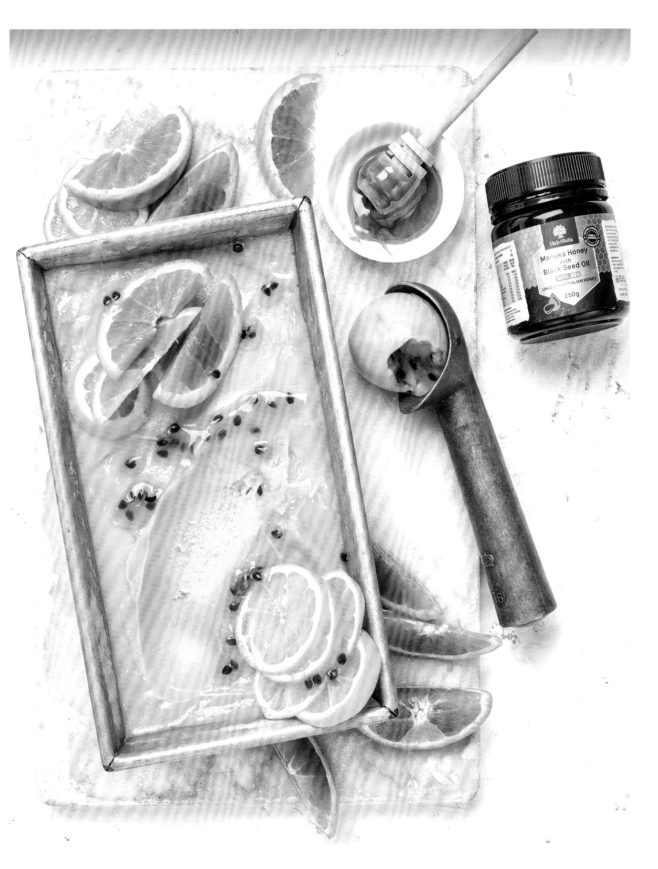

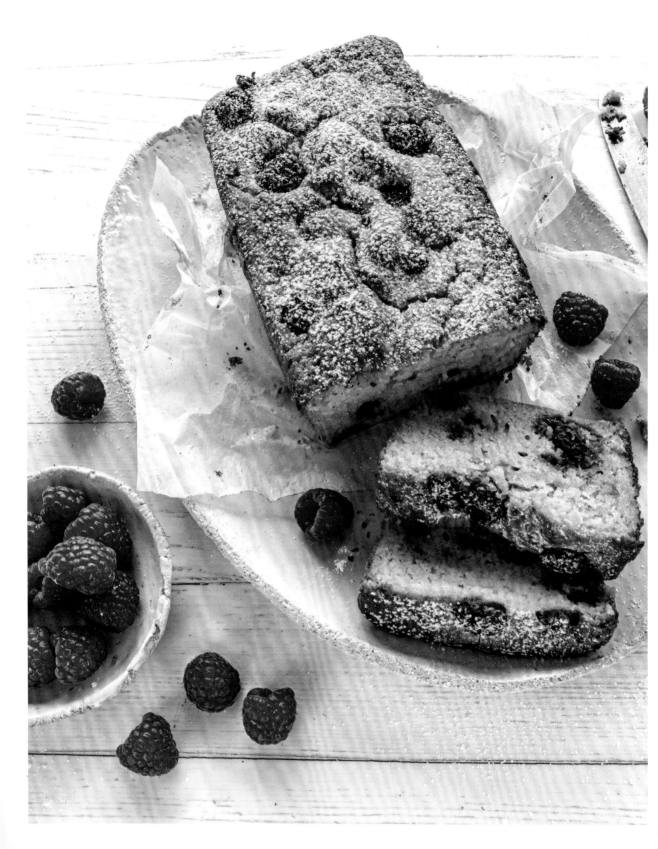

Raspberry slice

Gluten free • vegetarian • low carb • high protein • high fibre

SERVES: 8
PREP: 5 minutes
COOK: 30 minutes

Ingredients

1 cup almond meal

1 cup oat flour

1 scoop vegan protein powder

1 tablespoon baking powder

pinch of salt

⅔ cup maple syrup

1 cup kefir

½ cup coconut oil, melted

3 eggs, lightly beaten

½ cup frozen raspberries

Method

With the rack in the middle position, preheat the oven to 180°C.

Combine the dry ingredients in a bowl and set aside. Combine the wet ingredients in another bowl. Add the wet mix to the dry ingredients and gently stir with a spatula, until combined. Add the raspberries and stir gently.

Bake in a loaf tin for 30 minutes or until a skewer comes out clean.

Tip

Want a vegan version? Sub the eggs for one banana or 2 tablespoons of apple sauce, and the kefir for soy yoghurt.

Lemon seed muffins

Gluten free • vegan• low carb • high protein • high fibre

Ingredients

¼ cup coconut oil

¾ cup soy milk

8 tbsp freshly squeezed
     lemon juice

2 tbsp lemon zest

½ cup maple syrup

1 tsp vanilla extract

3 tbsp black nigella seeds

2 cups almond meal

½ cup oat flour

1 scoop vegan protein
     powder

1 tbsp baking powder

1 tsp bicarb (baking) soda

Method

Preheat oven to 180°C. Line a muffin tray with muffin papers.

Place the coconut oil in a bowl and microwave for 1 minute until melted. Add the rest of the ingredients and mix well, adding a splash of milk if too dry.

Divide the mixture between the muffin papers.

Bake in the oven for 15–20 minutes until risen or until a skewer comes out clean.

Tip

Want a keto-friendly version? Sub the maple syrup for monkfruit extract and omit the oat flour.

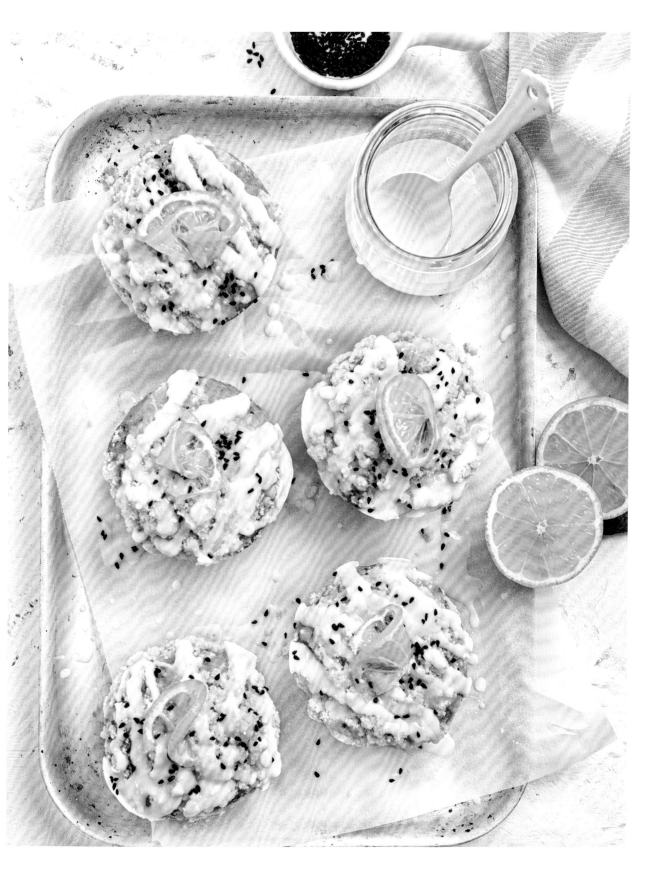

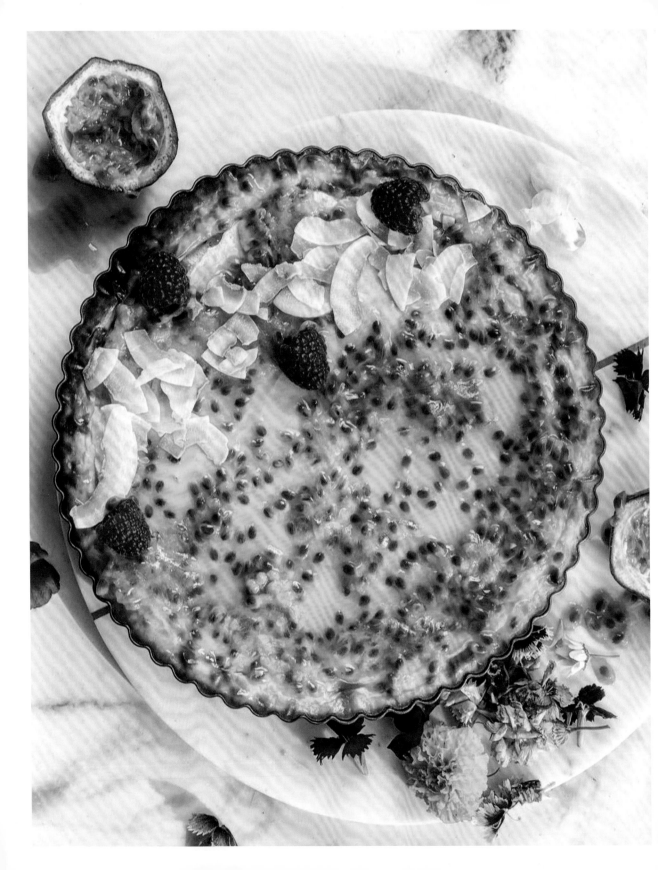

Passionfruit cheesecake

Gluten free • vegan • low carb • high protein • high fibre

Ingredients

2 cups almond meal

100 g vegan butter, melted

500 g vegan cream cheese

300 g vegan sour cream

½ cup silken tofu

½ cup maple syrup

½ cup passionfruit pulp

1 tsp vanilla bean paste

passionfruit and coconut
flakes, to serve

Method

Preheat the oven to 160°C.

Process the almond meal and butter in a food processor, then line a 30 cm springform cake tin with the mix.

Clean the food processor bowl then process the cream cheese, sour cream, tofu, maple syrup, passionfruit pulp and vanilla paste until smooth and creamy.

Pour the mix into the shell. Bake for 50 minutes. Allow to cool and refrigerate overnight.

To serve, top with more passionfruit and toasted coconut flakes.

Tip

Rather a non-vegan version? Use real cream cheese and sour cream and sub the tofu for two eggs.

Protein mocha pops

Gluten free • vegan • low carb • high protein • keto-friendly

SERVES: 6
PREP: 6–8 hours

Ingredients

4 scoops vegan protein powder

1 shot espresso coffee

640 ml soy milk

Method

Put all the ingredients in a food processor or blender on high. Pour into popsicle moulds and freeze overnight. Dust with a little raw cacao powder before serving.

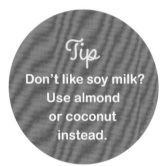

Tip
Don't like soy milk? Use almond or coconut instead.

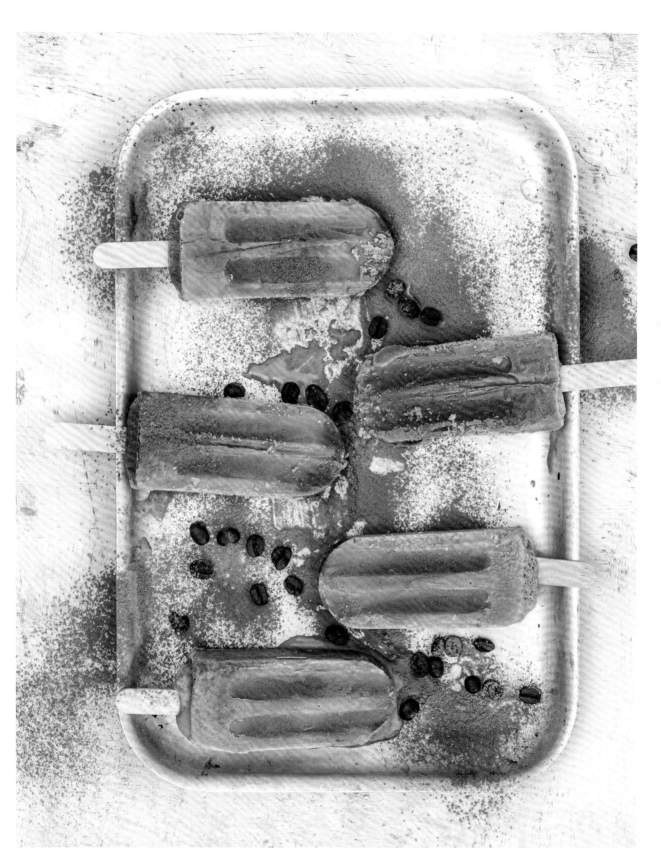

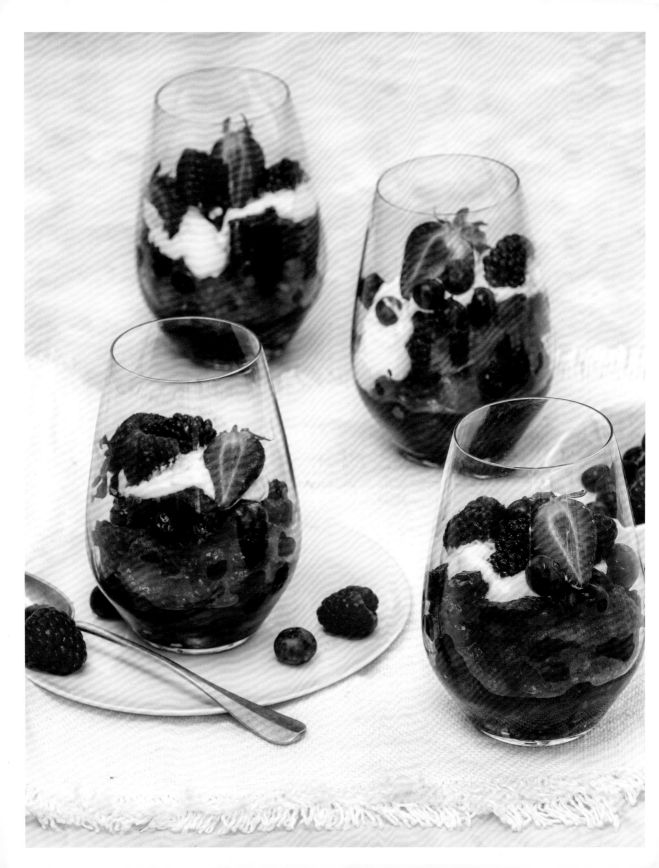

Gluten-free summer puddings

Gluten free • vegan • low carb

SERVES: 6
PREP: 6–8 hours

Ingredients

melted vegan butter,
    to grease

500 g mixed berries

40 g monkfruit sweetener

2 tbsp lemon juice

10 slices gluten-free bread,
    crusts removed

coconut yoghurt and
    extra berries, to serve

Method

Brush a pudding basin with melted butter and line the base with two to three layers of plastic wrap.

Put the berries monkfruit sweetener and lemon juice in a large saucepan and cook for about 5 minutes, until mixture is syrupy.

Line the basin with seven slices of gluten-free bread, allowing them to overlap. Press the bread together to seal making sure that the pudding basin is completely covered.

Reserve two-thirds of the berry mixture and set aside. Pour the rest of the mixture into the pudding basin and cover with remaining slices of bread. Place a plate over the top of the pudding and a weight on top of the plate. Refrigerate overnight or for at least eight hours.

When you're ready to serve, turn the pudding over onto a large serving plate and pour over the reserved berry mixture. Top with some fresh berries.

Serve in glasses with a dollop of coconut yoghurt.

Tip

After a keto-friendly version? Make my low carb fluffy bread rolls in a bread tin and use slices of that instead.

Low-carb black forest cake

Gluten free • vegan • low carb • high protein

SERVES: 8
PREP: 5 minutes
COOK: 20 minutes

Ingredients

2 cups almond flour

1 scoop vegan protein powder

1 tsp baking powder

1 cup raw cacao powder

½ teaspoon Himalayan pink salt

1 cup maple syrup

½ cup coconut oil, melted

½ cup coconut yoghurt

1 tin chickpea water (aquafaba), whipped

2 teaspoons vanilla extract

400 g coconut yoghurt

200 g jar sugar-free cherry jam

whipped coconut cream plus a handful of fresh cherries to serve

Method

Preheat oven to 180°C. Grease and line two round 20-cm cake tins.

Put all the dry ingredients in a large bowl and mix well to remove any lumps. Once combined, mix through the maple syrup, coconut oil, yoghurt, aquafaba and vanilla extract until a smooth batter forms.

Divide the batter between the cake tins and bake for 30–35 minutes. Leave the cakes to cool.

Whisk the coconut yoghurt using an electric whisk for around 5–10 minutes.

Once the cakes are cool, spread a layer of jam over one cake, then a layer of coconut cream over the top. Top with the second cake and repeat. Finish with fresh cherries and a swirl of cherry jam.

Tip

Want a keto-friendly version? Use half a cup of monkfruit sweetener instead of maple syrup.

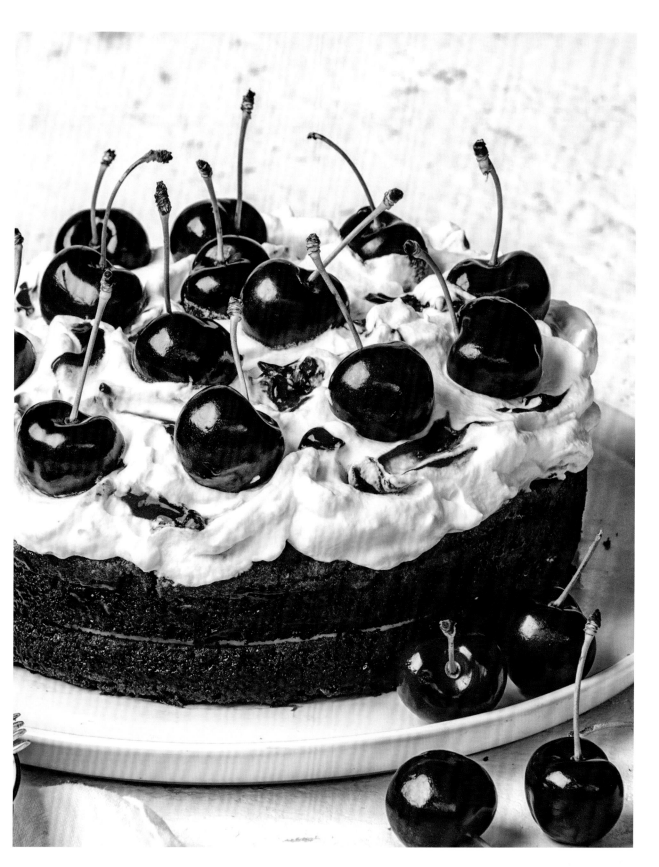

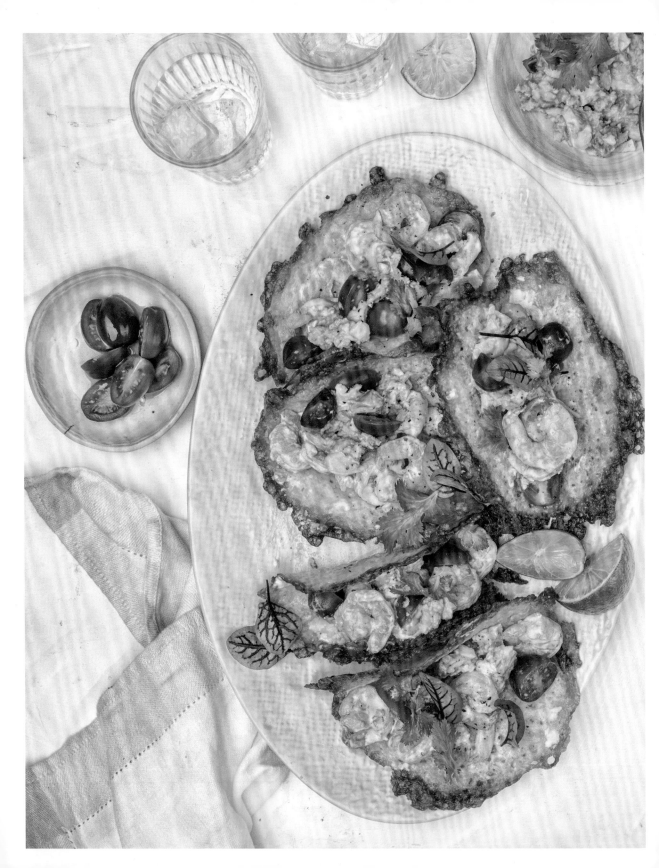

Parmesan prawn tacos

Gluten free • low carb • high protein • keto-friendly

SERVES: 2
PREP: 5 minutes
COOK: 20 minute

Ingredients

1 cup grated parmesan cheese

¼ tsp smoky paprika

150 g peeled prawns

1 tbsp butter

2 garlic cloves, crushed

½ tsp chilli flakes

salt and pepper, to taste

½ cup sour cream

zest and juice of 1 lime

3 tbsp freshly chopped coriander

½ an avocado, diced

½ cup cherry tomatoes, quartered

Method

Preheat the oven to 220°C. Line a baking tray with baking paper.

Combine the parmesan cheese and paprika and form six piles on the baking tray. Leave plenty of space between each pile so they don't stick together. Bake for about 8 minutes or until the cheese is melted, bubbling and golden brown.

Remove from the oven and let sit for about 2 minutes to cool. Peel away the cheese tacos and hang on a rolling pin on a wedge between an upside down muffin tin to create a taco shape. Leave to set for about 5 minutes.

Meanwhile, fry the prawns in the butter with the garlic and chilli flakes until cooked through and nice and pink. Add the seasoning and let cool for about 5 minutes.

Mix in the sour cream, lime juice, zest and coriander.

Fill the taco shells with the prawn mixture and top with avocado and cherry tomatoes.

Tip

Want a veggie version? Sub the prawns for tempeh.

173

SWEETS AND SNACKS

Kefir sorbet

Gluten free • vegan • low carb • high protein
• keto-friendly

SERVES: 6
PREP: 6–8 hours

Ingredients

½ cup lemon juice

2 tbsp lemon zest

½ cup monkfruit extract

6 to 8 sprigs fresh thyme

2 cups kefir

Method

Combine the lemon juice, zest, sugar, and thyme in a saucepan over medium heat. Cook until the sugar dissolves, about 3 to 5 minutes. Remove from the heat and let cool to lukewarm then stir in the kefir.

Chill the sorbet mixture in the fridge for at least 4 hours, or in the freezer for an hour before churning in an ice-cream maker. Churn until it resembles soft serve.

Transfer the sorbet to a freezer-safe container and flatten with the back of a spoon. Cover with plastic wrap and freeze until firm or overnight.

Soften at room temperature for a few minutes before serving.

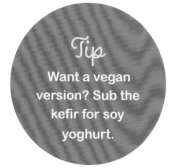

Tip

Want a vegan version? Sub the kefir for soy yoghurt.

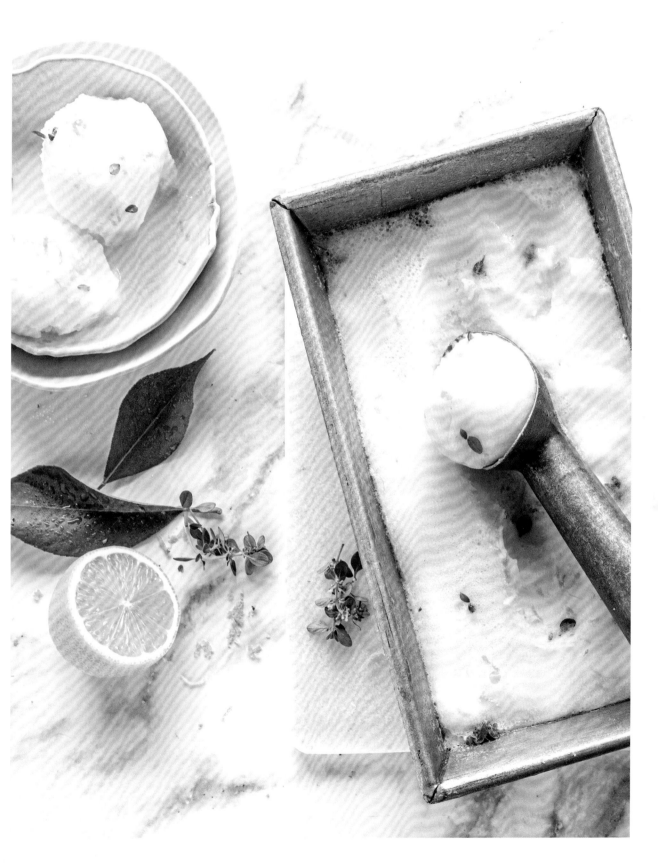

Footnotes

1 pubmed.ncbi.nlm.nih.gov/32329636/

2 www.ncbi.nlm.nih.gov/pmc/articles/PMC7468767/

3 obgyn.onlinelibrary.wiley.com/doi/10.1111/1471-0528.17290?af=R

4 www.ncbi.nlm.nih.gov/pmc/articles/PMC5728369/

5 www.sciencedaily.com/releases/2011/03/110331104053.htm

6 www.sciencedaily.com/releases/2011/03/110331104053.htm

7 pubmed.ncbi.nlm.nih.gov/30363011/

8 www.ncbi.nlm.nih.gov/pmc/articles/PMC4621258/

9 pubmed.ncbi.nlm.nih.gov/25051286/

10 www.ncbi.nlm.nih.gov/pmc/articles/PMC6892284/

11 www.ncbi.nlm.nih.gov/pmc/articles/PMC5731843/

12 www.ncbi.nlm.nih.gov/pmc/articles/PMC3257681/

13 www.ahajournals.org/doi/pdf/10.1161/01.HYP.0000218857.67880.75

14 www.ncbi.nlm.nih.gov/pmc/articles/PMC5643776/

15 www.ncbi.nlm.nih.gov/pmc/articles/PMC3270074/

16 www.menopause.org.au/hp/information-sheets/calcium-supplements

17 www.racgp.org.au/getattachment/631e40c5-1ce1-4da9-aeec-9c0b1ff1a515/attachment.aspx

18 www.eatforhealth.gov.au/nutrient-reference-values/nutrients/magnesium

19 www.ncbi.nlm.nih.gov/pmc/articles/PMC3195360/

20 www.ncbi.nlm.nih.gov/pmc/articles/PMC6372850/

21 pubmed.ncbi.nlm.nih.gov/30681787/

US $19.99

UK £14.99

First published in 2023 by New Holland Publishers
Sydney

Level 1, 178 Fox Valley Road, Wahroonga, NSW 2076, Australia

newhollandpublishers.com

A record of this book is held at the National Library of Australia.

ISBN 9781760795924

Text: Faye James
Photography: Darrin James
Recipe development: Faye James
Styling: Annette Forrest

Managing Director: Fiona Schultz
Project Editor: Liz Hardy
Designer: Andrew Davies
Production Director: Arlene Gippert

Printed in China

10 9 8 7 6 5 4 3 2 1

Keep up with New Holland Publishers:
 NewHollandPublishers
 @newhollandpublishers